"*The 90-Day Fitness Challenge* is a wonderful compilation of the principles, anecdotes and information that not only helped to change the lives of my friends, Phil and Amy Parham, but can serve to change the lives of its readers as well. From their DREAM principle to the daily mini-challenges and tips, along with the combination of faith principles, inspirational quotes, and noteworthy statistics, Phil and Amy provide guidance for anyone looking to get on the path to a healthy lifestyle."

—Bill Germanakos, winner, Season 4 of *NBC's The Biggest Loser*

"*The 90-Day Fitness Challenge* is a great read for those desiring to lose weight and keep God at the center. Having watched Phil and Amy work out at D1, I believe their testimony will motivate and inspire people to desire to better themselves. I have been around the fitness industry a long time and have a strong passion for overall wellness. It is awesome to experience Phil and Amy sharing a similar passion!"

—Will Bartholomew, president and CEO,
D1 Sports Training and Therapy

"Phil and Amy Parham prove there are no quick fixes, but in *The 90-Day Fitness Challenge*, they show how in a brief period of time you can lay the foundation for a lifetime of healthy habits."

—Brandi Koskie, DietsInReview.com

"Phil and Amy Parham inspired me on *The Biggest Loser*, and they will inspire you to reach your goals. This book covers aspects of health that so many others leave out. I was excited to get to the next chapter!"

—Danny Cahill, winner, Season 8 of *NBC's The Biggest Loser*

"The first book that I've ever read that clearly spells out the right steps to take to gain a healthy lifestyle. Phil and Amy Parham have taken the guess work out of the equation. Apply these principles and in 90 days your DREAM will be a reality."

—Rob Dempsey, morning radio DJ and multisport athlete

"It takes a special kind of courage to face your personal demons, and an even greater courage to accept that many of them exist as a result of your bad choices. The ultimate courage is to right those wrongs. Phil and Amy Parham have done just that, and their book will inspire many of us to do the same."

—Bill Ellis, morning radio host, "Ellis and Bradley Morning Show"

"Being on *The Biggest Loser* was one of the most significant times in my Christian life. God designed and desires us to be spiritually and physically healthy, and the impact on our lives is huge. Phil and Amy Parham are the only ones to have put into writing what so many former contestants now know—that weight loss, pursuing health, and becoming the person God intended us to be is not just an exercise program, but a faith journey as well. As a pastor and weight-loss group leader, I love that *The 90-Day Fitness Challenge* is a complete program, tying together amazing teaching and resources on changing to a healthy lifestyle while honoring and involving our Creator. This is THE book to get for individuals or groups looking to change their lives for the long term!"

—Rev. Matthew McNutt, contestant,
Season 3 of *NBC's The Biggest Loser*

"Phil and Amy Parham's *The 90-Day Fitness Challenge* is more than your typical diet book. They don't just *tell* you how to achieve long-lasting change in your life; they *show* you how to do it. Their story is inspiring, and their enthusiasm for good health and fitness is contagious. If you're looking for a practical program that can help you transform your life through realizing the critical connection between the physical and the spiritual, then *The 90-Day Fitness Challenge* may be exactly what you're looking for."

—Julie Hadden, first runner-up and biggest female loser,
Season 4 of *NBC's The Biggest Loser*;
author, *Fat Chance: Losing the Weight, Gaining My Worth*

"If you've tried every diet out there and are finally open to adapting a new way of life that gives you a real chance for success, look no further than Phil and Amy Parham's *The 90-Day Fitness Challenge*. Chock-full of motivation, sound advice, and doable actions that will set you up for a lifetime of success, it's a must-have guide for health and happiness!"

—Devin Alexander, host of *Healthy Decadence* (FitTV) and
author of the *New York Times* bestselling *Biggest Loser* cookbooks

"Amy and Phil Parham will help you understand that nutrition and fitness is a lifetime journey...not a sprint."

—Dr. Rick Kattouf II, host of *Rx Nutrition*
DVDs and author of *Forever Fit*

THE 90-DAY FITNESS CHALLENGE

PHIL PARHAM
AMY PARHAM

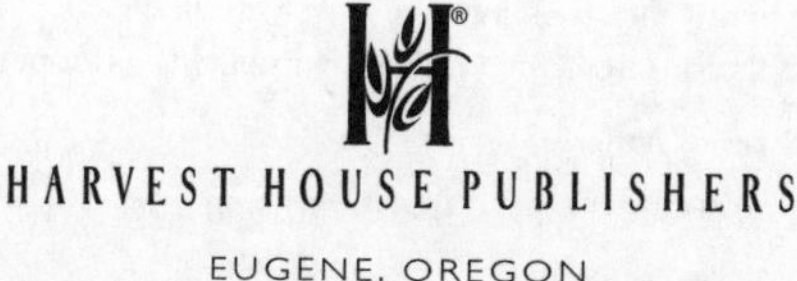

EUGENE, OREGON

Cover design by Dugan Design Group, Bloomington, Minnesota

Cover photo by Lauren N. Highsmith

Backcover author photo by Mitchell's Photography

Published in association with the literary agency Fedd & Company, Inc. Literary Agency (Esther Fedorkevich)

***The Biggest Loser* is not associated with this book or any of the views or information contained in this book.**

Readers are advised to consult with their physician or other medical practitioner before implementing the suggestions that follow. This book is not intended to take the place of sound medical advice or to treat specific maladies. Neither the authors nor the publisher assumes any liability for possible adverse consequences as a result of the information contained herein.

The 90-Day Fitness Challenge

Published by Harvest House Publishers
Eugene, Oregon 97402
www.harvesthousepublishers.com

Library of Congress Cataloging-in-Publication Data
Parham, Phil
The 90-day fitness challenge / Phil and Amy Parham.
p. cm.
ISBN 978-0-7369-2949-3 (pbk.)
1. Physical fitness. 2. Lifestyles. I. Parham, Amy, 1967- II. Title. III Title: Ninety-day fitness challenge.
RA781.P287 2010
613.7—dc22
2009047449

Printed in the United States of America

10 11 12 13 14 15 16 / BP-SK / 10 9 8 7 6 5 4 3 2 1

Contents

Acknowledgments

From Amy

From the time I was a little girl, I had the seed of a dream inside my heart to write a book. But just as a seed requires water to grow and develop, dreams require the guidance, support, and wisdom of many people to make them come true. I would like to thank the following people for their contribution in making this dream a reality...

My parents, Bill and Margaret Williams and Don Pearson; my siblings, Allyson Mauney, Donna Swett, and Matthew Williams; and my sister and brother-in-law, Joan and John Asher for their unconditional love and support. My children, Austin, Pearson, and Rhett, for the sacrifices they made to allow Mom and Dad to learn the lessons that we write about. Bob Harper, my "ranch" trainer, for showing me my strength. My "at home" trainer, D.J. Jordan, who was there for me closer than a brother every step of the way. Lolo, our assistant and adopted child, who has been a rock in turbulent times and the closest confidant. My friends, Carol and Tim Polin, who were truly friends and not just fans. Jennifer Miller and Phebe Simons for always being there to lend an ear. Todd Littleton, owner of LivN Nsidout Wellness Complex, and all of the people who sponsored and participated in our first "90-Day Fitness Challenge."

William Haynes for believing in us, encouraging us to do the first challenge, and helping us to see that writing a book was possible. All of our trainers at D1 Sports and Training who gave freely and never asked for anything in return. Many thanks go to our literary agent, Esther Fedorkevich, for her enthusiasm and support and to Amy Gregory for her patience and love for this project. To the cast and crew of *The Biggest Loser* season 6, who will forever hold a place of fond memories in our hearts.

Finally, to the love of my life, Phillip, who has remained a source of friendship, inspiration, and encouragement. Thank you for sticking with me for over twenty years. I love you!

From Phil

It's crazy to think that just over a year and a half ago I weighed 340 pounds, and now I'm finishing a weight-loss book. Life can really change on you! I would first start out by thanking God, who I believe has His hand on this project. You cannot look back at all the events that unfolded to see this book take shape and not see the divine hand of Providence.

I am so proud of our literary team. Esther, you are the greatest literary agent in the world! You are honest, you pull no punches, and most importantly you believe in Amy and me. Amy Gregory helped us with this manuscript, guided us through the process, and turned our words into magic. Amy, you are so patient and sweet. I looked forward to every call we had. I also thank Vivien, who does research and is such a blessing to work with. Special thanks to Dina White, who does publicity for us. Dina, you are amazing! To think we get to work with someone of your caliber still thrills me. You also are one of the believers. We feel it and appreciate all you do for us. We also are excited to be with Harvest House Publishers. We love all the gang there and hope this is the first of many successful projects we get to share together.

I thank my kids, Austin, Pearson, and Rhett. I love you boys! This process has been hard on you at times, and Mommy and Daddy know that. You guys are troopers, and we love you and cannot begin to tell you how proud we are of each one of you. I especially thank my sister Joan and brother-in-law John. They sacrificed with us and watched our kids for three months. They took care of everything, and I had no worries. Joan, you are the best sister a guy could have.

I want to shout out to everyone who encouraged us and helped us in this process. To our friend and assistant, Lolo, you are our family and we love you. To all my friends and family who believed in us and helped us—there are too many of you to mention, but you know who you are. We love you!

My friend Darren Anderson, who played racquetball with me and encouraged me every day. My trainer, D.J. Jordan, who is one of the best trainers in the world. You are awesome! My friends at D1 Sports and Training, we love you guys. You kick our behinds every day, and we love you for it. I am honored to have had two of the best trainers in America, Bob Harper and Jillian Michaels. I learned things from each of these masters and will remember it always.

A special thank-you is reserved for William Hayes, who had the vision for the first "90-Day Fitness Challenge." William, I want you to know how valuable you were to getting this book written. Many lives will be touched by your initial vision. You are truly a special person.

Thanks to my friend Tim Polin for his wonderful recipes in this book. You are a great friend. Also, thanks to Jeff Dumpert of Scratch Meals (scratchmeals.com) for giving me inspiration and your wonderful hummus recipe. You practice what you preach, and I admire you very much.

And finally I want to end with the love of my life, my wife, Amy. You are the most talented, beautiful, graceful, and wonderful woman I have ever known. To think I have been able to be united in marriage with you for over twenty years blows my mind. This has been one of the best experiences of my life, and we did it together! You are the absolute best thing that has ever happened to me. I love you always!

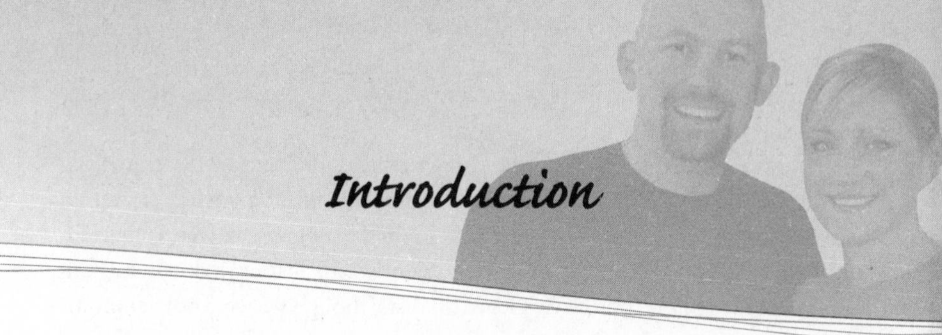

Introduction

Amy's Story

Six years ago, I was lying on my couch, gazing through an opening in the ceiling that led to the attic. My eyes slowly became fixated on a wooden beam. I began to wonder: *What would it feel like if I hung myself? Could the beam support my weight? How would I do it?* My downward spiral into a deep depression had reached the bottom. I felt completely hopeless and began to contemplate a permanent way out. How in the world did I allow myself to get to this point?

In four years, I had given birth to three sons, Austin, Pearson, and Rhett, and had gained seventy pounds. My body and spirit sagged under the extra weight. In 2003, Rhett was diagnosed with autism. As any mother who has high hopes and dreams for her children, I struggled with the diagnosis and dedicated much of my time and energy into finding ways to fix Rhett. I was physically exhausted and emotionally drained. I coped by binge eating every night. At the same time, my husband's business had collapsed, and we found ourselves under incredible financial pressure.

Every day felt like hell on earth. I would make myself get out of bed each morning, even though I didn't feel like it. One day I was praying, as I always did, for some guidance on how to fix Rhett. I was obsessed with finding a miracle cure because I couldn't accept that he wasn't going to be normal. In the depths of my spirit I heard God say, "Amy, you are not perfect and I love you. Why does Rhett have to be perfect for you to love him?" Instantly I felt a burden lift off my shoulders as I realized that if I would just love my little boy and trust God, He would take care of my son. This was the first step of my journey to get my life back on track.

Though the road was unbelievably long and hard at times, eventually the financial part of our lives and the challenges of having a child with autism began to straighten out. I knew that our weight was the last frontier to conquer. One night in 2008, having reached clinical obesity at 229 pounds, I was sitting on the sofa eating ice cream, crying, and watching *The Biggest Loser*. I suddenly decided to look on NBC.com to see what the process was for getting on the show.

A few months later, on Valentine's Day weekend, Phil and I were in Atlanta for the auditions. Though we were hopeful, we didn't hear anything from the network until two and a half months later. From the moment we were contacted until we were actually on the show was a whirlwind. Before we knew it, Phil and I were on a plane to Los Angeles as finalists, though we were not yet promised a slot on the show. The next week, Bob Harper, one of the show's fitness trainers, surprised us at our home to announce that out of 300,000 applicants, we were chosen for Season 6 of *The Biggest Loser*. Tears flowed down my face, and I remember thinking that this was the last piece of the puzzle to getting our lives back. There was no turning back.

Phil's Story

Even though I was an overweight child, I never let it stop me from becoming a success in business and being able to support my family. In 2004, however, my mortgage broker business went to pieces after my business partner left. It was a shock to my ego and a crushing blow to our bank accounts. My family lost not only our luxurious lifestyle but also our security. For the first time in my life, I was at a loss about what to do. My weight slowly began to creep up the scales, but I wasn't paying attention to it that much. I was too busy trying to formulate a plan on how to get my family out of debt. My health was the last thing on my mind.

I had no choice but to turn this devastating situation over to God about the same time my wife also surrendered. We knew that with Him, there had to be a way out of the pressure. Slowly but surely our lives started to turn around. My wife and I found new careers in real estate. We became the top sales agents, selling over sixty homes in our first year. We also found a new therapy for Rhett that helped him improve his language and behavior. While we were both feeling more inspired and motivated, Amy and I were still too busy with our family and new careers to give much thought to our health. Pushing forty, constantly feeling out of breath, and struggling to maintain my energy level, I knew it was only a matter of time before I had to do something about my weight. The one area I had ignored my whole life would now become my most important battleground.

I was at my heaviest, a staggering 340 pounds, when my wife took a step toward change and applied for both of us to be contestants on *The Biggest Loser*. There we began a new chapter of transforming our bodies—the only part of our lives holding us back from fulfilling all of our dreams. In only seven months, we together lost over 250 pounds, putting me at a trim 180 pounds and Amy at a svelte 124 pounds. We still have one of the highest percentages of weight loss of any couple in *The Biggest Loser*'s history.

Today

We've maintained our healthy weight as we've incorporated permanent lifestyle changes we learned on *The Biggest Loser*. Not only have we continued to be successful in our real estate business, but we are sharing with others the power of transforming health. The most life-changing lesson we've learned on our journey is that our success is only a small part of the big picture to inspire others. By living out our dreams, we are dedicated to helping others also live out their dreams.

When we got home from "the ranch," the place we went to for the program's highly intense exercise and nutrition regimen, we not only witnessed an outpouring of love and support, but we also got asked a lot of questions about how we changed our health so dramatically. Our good friend William Hayes suggested we get local sponsorship and plan an event to instruct and encourage others to take the same journey. So we took another step of faith and created the "90-Day Fitness Challenge," a program designed to help others lose weight and gain health in ninety days based on how we did it ourselves.

With much running around, making countless phone calls, and tending to last-minute details, we put together our first event in less than two weeks at LivN Nsidout Wellness Complex in Simpsonville, South Carolina, on January 7, 2009. Almost one thousand people showed up from five states. We were blown away at how magical the event turned out. When we saw how many people wanted to learn more about healthy living and losing weight, we put a mailing list together and sent out daily emails to these folks. We offered tips, encouragement, and pointed them in the right direction to better living. As weeks and months went by, the reports we got back were astounding. We received email after email from people who lost weight guided by what they learned in the "90-Day Fitness Challenge." Not only did the pounds drop, but many of these wonderful people experienced other life changes—some quit smoking, some mended their marriages, and others gained the courage to pursue lifelong dreams.

At the end of ninety days, we had a finale party sponsored by several local businesses. It was amazing to see the transformation of the people who had attended the initial event three months earlier. Those who had come to that first meeting depressed were now excited. Those who were unhealthy were now healthy. Those who felt tired, sluggish, and unmotivated were now energized, inspired, and motivated. It was an emotional and powerful experience for us, far beyond what words can say. These beautiful people reminded us of our own transformation.

We knew that God wanted to get this message out to more than just those folks, so we got involved with online communities, churches, corporations, and other organizations all across the United States. We traveled all over the country conducting "Challenge" events and saw a tremendous need for a book that will safely guide people to lose weight. We have been blessed to be a part of giving people a chance to reclaim their life by bettering their health. We hope to do the same for you with this book.

In *The 90-Day Fitness Challenge*, we will unfold the fundamentals of weight-loss through what we call the DREAM principle and by daily doses of encouragement and instruction for ninety days. The first five chapters will unpack our model of better health based on the five keys we believe are the most important to lose weight:

Dream about what you want your life to be

Recognize where you are today

Eat to live

Activate your body

Make a difference in the lives of others

Next, we will walk together with you through ninety days of your weight-loss journey by offering inspiration, motivation, and practical life skills through our daily challenge. We will include stories from our own lives, weight-management skills and tips learned from our experience on the show, and motivational weight-loss stories of those who have been inspired by our success.

Are you tired of making excuses for your weight? Are you tired of how terrible you feel? Are you tired of putting your life on hold because you are overweight? Do you want more energy? Do you want to feel good? Do you want to be healthy? Do you want to be motivated? Do you want to be challenged? Do you want to be inspired? Do you want to experience lifetime change?

I know you do and now is your time.

Are you ready to get started?

Part 1

The 90-Day Fitness Challenge DREAM Principle

1

Dream About What You Want Your Life to Be

A Word from Amy

As children our dreams seem limitless. I remember as a young girl climbing the dogwood tree in the yard of my house and hanging upside down on the branches, dreaming about what I wanted to be when I grew up. As I played, I told myself stories of all the great things I would do one day. I designed my dream house in my imagination. I imagined I would be a famous singer and, along with my sisters, put on pretend concerts using hairbrushes as microphones and the fireplace hearth as a stage. Like most girls, we also acted out our dream weddings. We wrote lists that detailed the colors of our bridesmaid dresses and the kind of flowers that would be in our bouquets. It was easy for me to dream and believe that all things were possible. I thought I could do anything, and nobody could tell me otherwise.

Think back to your own childhood. You probably had no trouble telling someone what you wanted to be when you grew up. Maybe it made complete sense to say you were going to be a country music singer or the president of the United States or a doctor (and maybe all at the same time). But guess what? What happened to me probably happened to you. We grew up. Life happened. And suddenly our dreams began to grow farther and farther out of our reach.

What About Me?

With all the responsibilities that come with having jobs, families, and being involved in our communities, churches, and schools, before we know it we have put everyone and everything else before our dreams. But wait. Isn't that the right thing to do? Shouldn't we always fill a need if we see it? Shouldn't we be less selfish and focus on someone or something other than ourselves?

How many times have you found yourself saying something like: If no one else will volunteer, maybe I should. If no one else will host the party, maybe I should. If no one else will bring the cupcakes, maybe I should. If no one else will work late, maybe I should.

We say these things to ourselves so often that our needs and wants get kicked to the wayside. Go back to school? Get a new job? Focus on our health? We convince ourselves it's not the right time. We'll do those things after we finish a particular project or when our kids start going to school or when our spouse gets promoted. But guess what? Even when that "right time" comes, we will have even more things to do than before. And we never end up taking care of ourselves the way we need to.

I know a little bit about this. For many years, I was an expert at always putting myself last. I could never say no to anyone. Saying no to someone meant that person may not like me, and I could not bear the thought of not pleasing everyone. The problem with being a people-pleaser is that you lose yourself. You become a different person. You turn into someone you think everyone else wants you to be. My family saw firsthand how depressed I became as I abandoned my needs and wants in order to look perfect in the eyes of others. They saw how exhausted I became and endured plenty of my meltdowns.

I remember one people-pleasing instance in particular. We were shuffling back and forth to doctors and specialists trying to get our son Rhett evaluated for what was eventually diagnosed as autism. It was a horrible time, and I felt as though the world was caving in on me.

One bright spot in this dark picture was a woman I met. She and I hit it off and quickly became very close friends. After a little while, she started working for my husband's business.

This friend of mine didn't have anyone who could pick up her kids at school in the afternoons, so I volunteered to do it for her. No big deal, right? Well, this all happened in the beginning stages of Rhett's autism where he screamed nonstop, especially when he was in the car. His screaming was so bad, I bought our other children earplugs because I was worried it would affect their hearing. I actually lost some hearing in my left ear because Rhett sat behind me in the car.

Our afternoon routine was the same every day. I would pack up Rhett in the car to go pick up my two other kids and hers at their school, which was an hour away. Rhett screamed the entire way. Then we would wait in the elementary school car line for thirty minutes for the kids to get let out. Rhett screamed while we waited. Once the three kids got in the car, we would all drive to the middle school to pick up my friend's daughter. More screaming. It was torture for the kids and me. Finally, we would drive an hour back home, and all the kids would stay at my house until my friend picked her children up.

It was months before I finally told my friend that I couldn't do it anymore. You know what happened? She wasn't upset at all. She was fine with me stepping down and had no trouble finding a replacement driver. I was so worried that she would be mad at me that I kept saying yes just to please her.

Does this scenario sound familiar? How many times have you sacrificed your time, your energy, your sanity, your health, or your relationships to do something to please someone else? When we do this, we simply endure our lives rather than live them.

Without dreams, we don't really live. We only exist. We go through the motions. We don't live the kind of life God has called each and every one of us to live.

In 2004, I found myself trapped inside a world that I did not want and in a body that I hated. And while I was still doing everything for everyone other than me, I was just not able to make everyone happy all the time. I felt like a complete failure. The only thing that made me feel better was food, and I turned to it all the time for comfort.

Eating so much made me increasingly tired. I remember the day that I stopped going upstairs in our home. There were two reasons for this. First, going up the stairs always revealed some destruction that Rhett had done. He would color on the walls, smear feces all over the windows, take the bifold closet doors off the tracks and throw them on the floor, run the water and overflow the bathtub, and so on. You never knew what you were going to find when you went upstairs. So I opted not to find out and stayed on the first floor as much as possible.

Second, walking up the stairs made me extremely winded and hurt my legs. Not wanting to face the fact that my weight might be affecting my health, I chose to avoid the issue. I had good reasoning behind this. If I never went up the stairs, I would never feel winded. If I never felt winded, I didn't have to admit I had a problem.

I survived a good portion of this trying time using the strategy of avoidance. But it only took me further from the life I once dreamed of living.

God Is the Giver of Dreams

The Bible tells us that if we delight in God, He will give us the desires of our heart (see Psalm 37:4). I am not a preacher, but I always interpreted that passage to mean that when we were created, along with God giving us our fingers and toes, He placed in our hearts a desire for fulfilling a specific purpose.

Desire propels us to push toward doing what we were created to do. It powers our dreams. It moves us in the direction of where we need to go. It makes us pursue someone to share our life with. It makes us long to have children. But desire can be minimized through tough circumstances. When life happens, it is easy to wake up one day and realize we have forgotten what it was that we dreamed about doing with our lives.

Think about your own desires and your current life circumstances. Have the desires of your heart gone away? Have you forgotten about the dreams of yesterday? Are you so consumed with life and its routines that you have no time or energy or even want to dream? What are those things you desire that you know, deep down in your heart, God has placed in you?

Before being a contestant on *The Biggest Loser*, I was not dreaming big dreams. I wasn't dreaming at all. I felt time slipping away from me as I struggled to fix all the financial problems that plagued our family while trying to figure out a way to best help Rhett. I was depressed. It took all the energy I had to get up in the morning. As soon as I got up, I prayed for God's strength to make it through another day.

God eventually answered my prayers. Day by day, the knots in my life slowly started to unravel. Phil and I became real estate agents and were making more money. We found a wonderful therapy for Rhett. We had a great group of friends and family. Things were looking up.

I've found that as soon as one area of my life gets straightened out, it gives me the courage to focus on other areas that need attention. The magnifying glass went full focus on our weight.

Through all the drama, trials, and troubles Phil and I experienced, we packed on the pounds. Phil was at his heaviest, a staggering 340 pounds, and I had reached clinical obesity at 229 pounds. My goodness, how were we going to get this weight off?

Once again, I believe that Providence stepped in. Who would have thought that the way God would plan for us to face this giant would be on a reality television show? But He did, and the things we learned forever changed the course of our lives.

The journey toward better health taught us that we needed to allow ourselves to wake up and dream again. God had more in store for us than even the wonderful things He was already doing with our family and our finances. He wasn't going to intervene in just one aspect of our lives; He wanted to work with us in every area so we could live lives of abundance. We had to stop settling and start dreaming.

It's Your Turn

You may be thinking that you have too many obstacles in your life. You may be thinking that you will never be able to overcome the challenges that face you in order to do the things you want to do. It is the dream that motivates the change. It is the dream that powers the desire. If you give yourself permission to start dreaming again, things will happen. Your life will change.

We want to take the first step with you in dreaming again. You need to start this journey by dreaming about what you want your life to be. Not whining about what it looks like right now. Not making excuses for why you can't change it. Not settling for a life that is mediocre. It's time to make a new vision for your life.

This book focuses on your health, and your dreams will revolve around that focal point. But don't stop there. Think about your personal life. Your career. Your family. Think about every facet of your life and the dreams that come from those places. It doesn't matter how big or small they are. What matters is that you just dream.

How do you do this? Start by finding a quiet place where you can spend a half hour or so alone without distractions. Take yourself back to the time when you believed that dreams could come true. Think about what your life could look like and how you would feel if some of your dreams came true. Maybe you want to lose fifty pounds. Maybe you want to pay off your debt. Maybe you want to be a better parent. Maybe you want to go back to school. The point of this exercise is to imagine a better life.

Here are some questions to help get you started. Ask yourself these questions out loud, and in the space below, write down your answers. You might want to create some of your own questions and answers.

"If I were at a healthy weight, what would that look like?"

"What would it feel like to buy clothes in size ____?"

"What if I didn't have to dread getting dressed in the morning?"

"What if I could play with my kids without getting out of breath?"

"What would I do differently if money were not an issue?"

"What churches or charities would I give to if I had more than enough finances?"

"If nothing were holding me back, what would I most like to do in life that I haven't done?"

"What things did I dream about doing before life took over?"

Dust off that box of dreams hidden deep within you and know that anything is possible with God. God has not forgotten you. He has bigger plans for you. Bigger than you can imagine. Make the commitment to dream, and it will keep you moving in the right direction even in your toughest times.

2

Recognize Where You Are Today

A Note from Phil

Dreaming is fun, isn't it? I hope you took the time in the last chapter to reflect on the deep desires of your heart. It is such an important first step in your new adventure of gaining better health and losing weight.

How did you feel when you read the title of this chapter? Perhaps you let out a big sigh or even groaned. Recognizing where you are today may not be a fun thing to think about. But it is something that we all must come to terms with before we take action to better our health. Step 2 of the DREAM principle requires us to admit that we are in a place we don't want to be and to see exactly what that place looks like in order to take the next steps.

Being honest about my health was a challenge for me. My life was spent making excuses and promises I couldn't keep. I had been severely overweight for a long time, but I figured if I never acknowledged that, then maybe it wasn't true. I lived much of my life avoiding the truth that was right in front of me—I was fat—and used many strategies to help me do this.

I avoided doctors because I did not want to hear what they might say. I went only when something was seriously wrong or I had an illness I couldn't shake. Knowing I was going to see a doctor scared me to death. In the back of my mind I had thoughts like: *Is he going to weigh me? I mean, I only have the flu. He shouldn't ask me about my weight, right?*

I stayed away from mirrors so I didn't have to face what I looked like. When I walked through our bedroom, I kept my eyes to the right to avoid the dresser mirror. I did the same thing when I walked into our bathroom. The mirror was on the left, so I averted my eyes to the right. When I made it to the closet, there was always a sigh of relief because there were no mirrors. I felt as if I had gone through a minefield to get to that safe place and I had, once again, survived. I did not realize the extent of all of these secret rituals until after I lost the weight. Avoiding mirrors had become second nature.

Another way I ignored my obesity was complaining about clothing stores that didn't carry enough larger sizes. Most of the chain stores didn't offer XXX sizes. I shopped at Walmart because they met my clothing needs, but I always left angry since I was charged two dollars more for the "Big and Tall" sizes. I felt insulted and discriminated against. It's funny how mad I was at the store when the real problem was me.

Reality Check

Some things weren't so easy to ignore. I remember one day I was sweating profusely and felt weird. In hindsight, I was showing signs of prediabetes, but at the time I had no idea what diabetes was. I was ignorant, and I now believe I was ignorant on purpose. I didn't want to acknowledge or accept what was happening to my health. Soon I began to wonder if something was seriously wrong with me. I suspected diabetes because I knew some people with similar medical problems who had the disease. I wondered how long I had before I needed to take insulin.

I was checking on a rental property one morning when the sweating happened again. I knew I had no choice. I pulled into a drugstore and bought a diabetes testing kit. I was so scared that I didn't even tell Amy about it. Although I bought it, I was too afraid to use it. I didn't want to face what it might say. So I hid the kit in the drawer of my desk. Later Amy found it and asked me about it. I think it freaked her out a little. Why was I so afraid? Why did I deny the truth? Why did I not think rationally about my physical problem? I am rational about so many things in my life, why not this?

I believe when it comes to our weight, we have a hard time being real. Do you feel the same way? When you come face-to-face with the number on the scale, what thoughts run through your mind? Do you feel like a failure? Do you think others will judge you? Do you think you'll be unable to get healthier? Do you think it makes you a bad person? Do you think you'll never be able to repair any damage?

Many folks who struggle with admitting where they are tend to hide from the truth. The reasons we do this are varied, but there is no denying that you need to properly assess where you are today to be able to move forward. I know it can be a tough process, but there are some practical action items you simply must do. (I'll talk about these in more detail toward the end of this chapter.)

You need to look in a mirror. You need to weigh yourself and get your measurements taken. You need to get a physical. You need to know what your blood pressure and blood sugar readings are. And you need to see these things in black and white so you have no choice but to admit where you are physically.

It might make you upset or sad, but I want to encourage you instead to get mad. Get mad at yourself for allowing things to go this far. Get mad at the unhealthy habits that you have allowed to control your life. Get mad at how you have put others before your own well-being. Then use that anger to make you stronger. Use that anger to inspire you. Use that anger to take action. You can face this giant. You *have* to face it. You and only you have the power to make a change in your life, but you've got to start now. Recognize where you are.

My Time of Change

Part of the process for applying for *The Biggest Loser* is getting a physical. You have to be overweight enough to go on the show, yet healthy enough to get through it. I was on the verge of many major health problems. I was desperate.

I didn't sleep well the night before my physical. My stress level was at an all-time high. I didn't want to know what the doctor had to say, though I think my subconscious really did. Deep down, I wanted to change, and I am so glad I was forced to get a physical. I was also required to meet with a nutritionist, who helped me identify my eating habits. As you can imagine, the results were not good.

While filming the first episode of the show, I met with Dr. Rob Huizenga, a weight-loss expert. We walked into a room, and on the wall was a projector screen. On the screen I saw a picture of my liver. The doctor told me that I had a fatty liver. Now, I knew that I had fat all over my body, but I never thought about my liver being fat too. Dr. H said that if I continued my indulgent lifestyle, my liver problem was going to get worse. Already my liver had deteriorated as if I had been an alcoholic all my life. I never realized that the fast food I had been gobbling up could wreak the same havoc as liquor.

There was more. My blood pressure was also very high, there was fat in my blood, and my heart was starting to become enlarged. These were all wake-up calls that told me I was going to have to change.

I remember holding Amy's hand and thinking about my kids and how I was a poor role model for them. Here I was, obese and sick, teaching them by my example to follow in my footsteps. They always said they wanted to be just like their dad, but their dad was looking pretty much like a failure. I broke down, and right then I vowed that I would change. I had been worried that I might not see my kids graduate or get married. Being forced to come to terms with my health meant that I would.

I think about the first weigh-in on the show. It was an emotionally charged event, one that I can't even describe. I, a man who avoided being shirtless in public at all costs because of how embarrassing it was to expose my body, stood in front of millions of people wearing nothing but a pair of shorts. Although I felt humiliated standing on that scale, it was worth it. I was exposed in every sense of the word. I couldn't hide any longer. It wasn't an option.

I remember looking at my wife and making the decision that saved my life. I told Amy I loved her, and then I asked her if she would let me focus on myself for a while. I needed to change. I was tired of being fat. I needed to better my health for me. As much as I loved Amy, I could not make this change because of her or because she wanted me to. I couldn't even change for the kids, as much as I loved them. And I certainly wasn't going to do this for any stranger or doctor. I had to do this for me. It was time for me to realize that I was worth it.

When we do our live "Challenge" events, we offer weigh-in and blood pressure stations so people can face these facts. We give them an opportunity to see where they are so they can start making their own changes.

Are you hiding from the facts? Are you turning a blind eye toward the truth—that your health is in bad shape—because the issue seems too overwhelming to confront? Today is the day to start looking in the mirror. Start seeing where you really are. Stop lying to yourself and acknowledge the truth. Know that you can change for the better.

We have work to do. Your life will not change until you make the decision to change it. The problem is not whether you have the power to change it, but whether you have made a decision to change it. Today, right now, make a commitment to yourself that you will be honest with yourself throughout *The 90-Day Fitness Challenge*. No more hiding. No more denying. No more ignoring. No more avoiding.

This is especially important right now. I'm going to give you a launching pad that you need to establish before you jump into the challenge. Are you ready to get started?

Things You Can Do Now to Recognize Where You Are

Space is available at the end of this chapter for you to chart your starting points (your initial weight, blood pressure reading, and so on). As you go through the following checklist, you might want to write down the numbers in the margin. Then when you're done, you can transfer them all to the spaces provided.

See a doctor. Schedule an appointment with your primary physician to get a physical. Your doctor will help you determine what, if any, medical problems you have as result of the extra weight and can help monitor your progress. I highly recommend having your doctor involved in recognizing the condition of your body in this initial part of the challenge. Make sure your doctor gives you a full physical and blood work. This is how he or she will gauge where you are. After ninety days, you won't believe the changes.

Get weighed. You can do this at your doctor's office during your physical. Find out what you weigh and how many pounds you have to lose to reach a realistic and healthy weight. Your goal should not be to "get skinny," but to maintain a weight that is healthy for your body. Also, as you continue to weigh yourself throughout the journey, do so at the same time, preferably in the morning. Our weight fluctuates throughout the day depending on our water and food intake. I always weigh myself right after I wake up.

Get your blood pressure reading. Your weight and your blood pressure are connected. The more pounds on your frame, the higher your blood pressure will be. That's a fact. Having high blood pressure, called hypertension, can result in all sorts of physical problems, such as stroke, heart attack, heart failure, and renal failure. This is serious business. Make sure your doctor checks this during your physical. Also, many pharmacies offer self-service blood pressure stations in their store. Anytime you want to find out what your blood pressure is, just walk into one of those places and find out.

Take your measurements. This is one of the best ways to measure your weight-loss progress. We all store and lose fat in different places in our body. Measuring yourself will give you a better idea of where you're losing fat. While the scale will tell you the amount of pounds lost, measuring your body will track where you've lost inches. There are a couple of ways you can do this. You can have your doctor measure you or, if you are a member of a gym, you can have a trainer measure you. You can even do this yourself with a tape measure. I highly recommend you get your measurements taken by a professional. However, if you opt to do this on your own, grab a cloth tape measure, a pencil, and follow these instructions.

- Get naked. This is the most accurate way of taking your measurements.
- Shoulders. Measure from one shoulder across in a straight line to the next, from largest point to largest point.

- Chest. Measure around the nipple line.
- Waist. Measure the narrowest part of your trunk, or approximately an inch or two above your belly button. Don't cheat and suck in your stomach!
- Hips. Put your heels together and measure the hips around the fullest part of your buttocks.
- Thighs. Measure the upper thighs, just below where your bottom meets the back of your thigh.

Find out your body mass index (BMI). BMI is based on a person's weight and height and is used to estimate a healthy body weight and to screen for weight categories that may lead to health problems. According to the Centers for Disease Control, a healthy BMI range is between 18.5 and 24.9. To figure out your BMI, use this formula:

$$\frac{\text{weight (lbs)} \times 703}{\text{height (in)}^2}$$

If you don't care to do the math, no worries. A number of online BMI calculators can do this for you (see the one provided by the Department of Health and Human Services at www.nhlbisupport.com/bmi/). Don't hesitate to ask your doctor or personal trainer to help you figure this out.

Find out your body fat percentage. This is the total weight of a person's fat divided by how much they weigh. This number includes both essential fat and storage fat. Essential fat is what is necessary to maintain life and reproductive functions. Because women have different levels of hormones than men and have the ability to bear children, their essential body fat percentage is higher than that for men. On average, men should keep about 2-5 percent of essential fat, women 10-13 percent. Storage fat consists of fat accumulation in adipose tissue, the parts that protect our internal organs.

Under the skin is a layer of subcutaneous fat. The percentage of total body fat is measured by taking a skinfold at different points in your body and measuring it with a pair of calipers. Once again, I suggest talking to your doctor or a trainer at the gym to help you do this.

Calculate your basal metabolic rate (BMR). Your BMR determines the number of calories you burn a day just by doing nothing. Even if you lie in bed all day, your body expends energy. The number decreases as you get older and your metabolism slows down, and it increases if you have more muscle mass and are active. This number is calculated by using your height, weight, age, and daily activity level. To lose weight, you must consume fewer calories (by eating less) or burn more (through exercise) than your BMR. Here is how you can calculate your BMR using a simple formula. If you don't want to do the math, just research "BMR calculators" online and use those tools to calculate it for you.

Step 1: Figure out your base formula

- Women: 655 + (4.3 x weight in pounds) + (4.7 x height in inches)−(4.7 x age in years)
- Men: 66 + (6.3 x weight in pounds) + (12.9 x height in inches)−(6.8 x age in years)

Step 2: Calculate your activity level

- If you are sedentary : BMR x 20 percent
- If you are lightly active: BMR x 30 percent
- If you are moderately active (you exercise most days a week): BMR x 40 percent
- If you are very active (you exercise intensely on a daily basis or for prolonged periods): BMR x 50 percent
- If you are extra active (you do hard labor or are in athletic training): BMR x 60 percent

Step 3: Add the activity level number to your BMR.
Again, to lose weight you'll need to take in fewer calories than this result.

Take a picture of yourself. This will be your official "before" picture. You will be amazed and encouraged to see how much your body has changed in ninety days. Wear a bathing suit in this photo and have a family member or friend take the picture for you. Make sure you get the front, back, and both sides. You can tape this to your refrigerator or put it in a more private place, such as the drawer of your desk. Just keep it where you can see it and let it motivate you on this challenge toward better health.

There are more things to do as it concerns eating and working out, and we'll cover those in the next two chapters. You'll be keeping a food journal of what you eat so you can see how many calories you regularly ingest, where some of your bad habits lie, and what your emotional triggers are. We'll also have you clean out your pantry of food that's bad for you, such as processed and artificial foods.

Before you learn about how to eat healthy and maintain those habits, let's talk about preliminary goal setting. In the section below, you need to write down the numbers we just talked about and, underneath that part, write in your goals based on your starting figures.

Be realistic. If your doctor tells you you need to lose thirty pounds, don't write in a weight-loss goal of fifty pounds. Make your goal healthy, realistic, and manageable. Your doctor or trainer can help you determine where you want to be.

No matter how bad you feel about where you are, it can get better. Your numbers can change. Your weight can decrease. Medical problems you may have can disappear.

Here are some of our numbers when we started and what they were at the end of the show (for me, it was a seven-month period).

Phil's Before Stats:	*Phil's After Stats*:
Age: 41	Age: 41
Weight: 326 lbs	Weight: 180 lbs
Body fat: 46%	Body fat: 17%
BMI: 48.7	BMI: 26.9

Amy's Before Stats:	*Amy's After Stats*:
Age: 40	Age: 40
Weight: 223 lbs	Weight: 124 lbs
Body fat: 54%	Body fat: 26%
BMI: 38.6	BMI: 21.5

I am so thankful that we have these records. When you get to the final page in this book and accomplish your goal of finishing the "90-Day Fitness Challenge," you will have the opportunity to write in your current stats. You're not going to believe the changes you made in your health and body.

Be encouraged. Be hopeful. Have faith. You *can* get where you want to be!

My Starting Point:

Today I weigh ______ pounds.

Today my blood pressure is _____/_____.

Today my BMI is _________.

Today I measure

_____ shoulders

_____ chest

_____ waist

_____ hips

_____ thighs

Today my BMR is _________.

My Goals:

By ___________ (date), I want to be _______ pounds.

By ___________ (date), I want my blood pressure to read _____/_____.

By ___________ (date), I want my BMI to be _________.

By ___________ (date), I want my measurements to be:

_____ shoulders

_____ chest

_____ waist

_____ hips

_____ thighs

At the end of this "Challenge," I want you to turn to appendix A to see how you did. There you can write in your old stats and the new stats and compare the difference. You will be amazed at your results.

We've got a lot of learning to do when it comes to what you put in your mouth. In the next chapter, you'll to learn how to eat, what to eat, when to eat, and the best and worst foods for you. Don't worry. Eating healthy is not boring or tasteless. We're going to make this as delicious for you as we can.

3

Eat to Live

A Note from Phil

Have you ever been on a diet? Since you are reading this book, the odds that you said yes are pretty good. The "90-Day Fitness Challenge" is not a diet; it's a lifestyle. The changes you will make and the information you will learn are things you will live by forever. Not just for ninety days.

We are here to make you informed about nutrition and to equip you to change your bad eating habits and misconceptions about food. Before I lost the weight, I used to think this was way too complicated. Just take a trip down the aisles of your favorite bookstore. Bookshelves are lined with diet books. One expert says this. Another expert says that. The amount of information out there is overwhelming.

Don't worry. We won't overwhelm you. If you know the basics about nutrition and eating to lose weight, you can grow and learn more from there. Just as you have established a starting point for where you are physically, this chapter is your launching pad for learning how and what to eat. From here, you will be able to make good decisions that will make permanent change happen.

Why Do We Eat?

The third key to our DREAM principle is *eating to live*. It's about reprogramming your mind to use food as fuel. Food is not meant to comfort you, to satisfy your cravings, or to be your best friend. It is meant to help your body run properly and efficiently. The Bible tells us that we are fearfully and wonderfully made (see Psalm 139). Your body is a wonderful, well-crafted machine meant to do good things. And that means you have to put good things into it.

Before I lost all this weight, I never thought too much about what I was eating. If it tasted good, I ate it. I also ate simply because I felt sad, happy, or bored. Now I have a different mentality and I am in control of what I eat. While I used to attach so much emotion to food, it does not have that power over me anymore. Also, I get to choose the foods that I know will make my body work better. I ask myself the right questions, such as "Are my food choices aiding or robbing me of health?" You can gain that same control. Every time you sit down to eat a meal or snack, you have to ask yourself whether it will fuel your body or slow it down. This is the mind game you have to conquer.

If you use food as a crutch or to fulfill some emotional need, stop. You have to renew your thinking. Sometimes you can't do this on your own. Find a counselor, a support group, or a professional who can help you overcome those underlying issues so you can relearn the proper way to look at food.

What Do We Eat?

Think Natural

The most important rule you need to learn about good nutrition is to choose foods that are natural, such as fresh fruits, vegetables, nuts, and lean meats. *Natural* means that the food is as close to its original state as possible and has not been or is only minimally processed. On the show, trainer Jillian Michaels often told us to think of it like this: when you choose a food item, does it have a mother or does it come from the ground? If the answer is yes, great. If not, don't eat it.

Why is this important? Your body functions at its best when nourished by natural foods. If you eat foods that have been chemically or otherwise altered, your body doesn't know how to properly process it. Did you know that many people are undernourished? It's not because they don't eat, but because they eat lousy fake food that does not properly feed their bodies.

Our bodies are efficient at healing themselves with the right foods. The more natural you eat, the less often you are sick. Americans are among the sickest people in the world. I believe it comes back to our diet. Many people in our country eat frequently at fast-food restaurants. All that preservative-filled food could be sending us to an early grave. It's time to stop eating fast food. Let's drive past the drive-thru.

I recently met a lady who had ovarian cancer ten years ago. She was diagnosed when the cancer was in stage III or IV, and she was told she had only a few months to live. She immediately had surgery, and the doctors removed as much of the cancer as they could. She was supposed to start chemotherapy right away, but she refused the treatment. She told the doctor, "Thanks, but no thanks," and instead made some radical changes to her diet.

She started eating only foods that were all natural. She juiced fruits and vegetables, which naturally boosted her immune system with a ton of vitamins and minerals. You know what happened? She started getting better even without chemotherapy. Today, this lady is alive and healthy.

I think about myself. When I started the program, I had a fatty liver, an enlarged heart, was prediabetic and, of course, grossly overweight. After only six weeks of working out regularly and eating natural foods, all my vitals were turned around (though I still needed to lose more weight). It's amazing what the right foods will do to your body.

Below is a list of foods Amy and I regularly eat that have helped us lose weight and keep it off. As you can see, these are all natural. Appendix B offers a more comprehensive shopping list that we use to choose our meals and snacks. We also provide you a seven-day meal plan in appendix C, but for most of the "Challenge," you will be responsible for planning your own meals.

Recommended Foods

Protein Sources

- eat only lean cuts of meat: chicken, turkey, fish, beef (sirloin or round cuts), lamb
- turkey sausage and bacon
- eggs
- vegetarian choices include firm tofu, tempeh, lentils, kidney beans, lima beans, black beans, chickpeas

Carb Sources

- oatmeal (not instant)
- fruits
- vegetables, vegetables, vegetables
- brown rice
- whole grains

Fat Sources

- olive oil (the best for cooking; use cold-pressed, extra virgin olive oil)
- safflower oil
- coconut oil (great for high-heat cooking)
- almond oil

- avocado
- nuts

Say Yes to Fiber

Never in my life had I given much thought to fiber. Sure, I saw commercials that told me fiber was important, but I didn't think it applied to me.

The American Dietetic Association recommends that we get twenty-five to thirty grams of fiber per day. Most Americans get about half that and, as a result, are constipated, have headaches, and generally feel tired and sluggish. Fiber is essential to good digestive health. If you get enough fiber in your diet, your bowels will move daily (which is ideal) and you'll feel better. Fiber absorbs large amounts of water in the bowels, which makes it easier for stools to pass through your system. When you have regular bowel movements, toxins are regularly released from your body, making you feel better and improving your overall health.

Getting enough fiber in your diet can decrease your risk of heart disease, cancer, diabetes, and kidney stones. Take a look at what you are eating this week and measure the amount of fiber in your diet. If you are eating less than twenty-five grams a day, it's not enough. Choose foods that are rich in fiber, such as fruits, vegetables, beans, and whole grain foods such as brown rice, whole wheat bread, and whole grain cereals (Fiber One and All-Bran).

Another easy way to add fiber is to eat ground flax seed. It tastes great as an addition to oatmeal or cereal. Start out with one teaspoon a day and work your way up slowly to two to four tablespoons. Make sure you grind the seeds before eating them so they don't just pass through your system. I use my coffee grinder and grind them right before I eat them.

Drink Your Water

Water is an essential component of good health because much of our bodies consists of it. If we don't drink enough, we become dehydrated and can get a whole slew of health problems. Here are just a few wonderful things drinking enough water does for you:

- Keeps your energy up
- Keeps your weight down
- Removes waste and eliminates toxins
- Helps carry nutrients and oxygen to cells

- Cushions joints
- Helps your body absorb nutrients
- Hydrates skin and hair
- Regulates body temperature

How much water is enough? You should drink half your body's weight (in pounds) in ounces of water each day. So if you weigh two hundred pounds, you should be drinking one hundred ounces of water. When Amy and I started our journey, we didn't drink enough water. When I committed to start drinking water, I remember feeling as though I couldn't get enough water, especially during my workouts. I was thirsty all the time because my body was trying to tell me I was dehydrated. I made the decision then to keep water with me at all times and drink it. I still do. I always carry a water bottle with me so I am never without it.

Here are some other things I do that help me stay hydrated all day. As soon as I get up in the morning, I drink sixteen ounces of water. This begins to flush out the toxins and get my body moving in the morning. I drink water with each meal and snack. I also drink before, during, and after a workout. I suggest for this challenge you commit to drinking only water. You should always be conscious of calories from beverages. Soda, fancy coffees, and even juices can pack on sugar and calories. Do your best to substitute water for all your drinks. I now love unsweetened tea and a small amount of black coffee. I will also drink the occasional cup of green tea. I am still amazed at how my cravings have left, my skin and overall appearance and general health have changed by incorporating the proper amount of water into my diet.

Make a conscious effort to drink more water, and your body will thank you for it.

Get Rid of Sugar

Unsweeten your tooth. So many people tell me, "Phil, I have a sweet tooth. I just can't help it." I tell them, "That's not true. You're just addicted to sugar." Sugar addiction is a huge problem in this country because sugar is everywhere. It's found in many of our foods and beverages. Just go through your pantry, pick a food item off the shelf, and read the ingredients label. Notice how many grams of sugar are in that product. I bet it's a lot.

When I started on the ranch, I was a borderline type 2 diabetic (non-insulin-dependent). Had I not secretly worried about it and stopped eating sweets,

I believe I would have become a full-blown diabetic. I thank *The Biggest Loser* for not having any sugar on the campus, which helped me change the course of my life.

Remember my first rule of eating? Sugar cane is natural, but refined sugar or high fructose sugar is not found in nature. They are highly concentrated, processed, and man-made products. I recommend you read the book *Sugar Blues* by William Dufty. It will open your eyes to the dangers of sugar and how it is a leading factor in depression and other medical problems.

Why would you want to sweeten your food with processed sugars when you can eat more natural foods and find better sweetener alternatives? Here are some natural sugar alternatives that have minimal to zero calories. Most grocery stores now carry these products, but some will be found in the pharmacy.

- Xylitol
- Stevia
- Truvia
- Local wildflower honey
- Agave nectar

My recommendation to you is to read labels. You will be astounded at all the sugar you find. It comes in many different names. It sneaks in everywhere. Here are some other possible code names for sugar:

- Corn sweetener
- Corn syrup or corn syrup solids
- Dehydrated cane juice
- Dextrin
- Dextrose
- Fructose (from fruit, we are not as concerned about)
- Fruit juice concentrate
- Glucose
- High-fructose corn syrup
- Honey
- Invert sugar
- Lactose

- Maltodextrin
- Malt syrup
- Maltose
- Maple syrup
- Molasses
- Raw sugar
- Rice syrup
- Saccharose
- Sorghum or sorghum syrup
- Sucrose
- Syrup
- Treacle
- Turbinado sugar
- Xylose

Remember your body does not care what it's called. It still sees it all as just "sugar."

Salt Be Gone

Salt is a dietary mineral mostly made up of sodium chloride. You need some sodium in your diet, but most people eat way too much. According to the USDA, we should consume no more than 2300 milligrams of sodium a day. A healthy range would be 1500-2300 milligrams a day. Yet the average American gets 3000-5000 milligrams of sodium each day. Way too much.

Here's what excess salt in your diet does:

- increases the number of fat cells in your body
- makes the fat cells you have get larger
- increases your insulin resistance
- makes you more hungry and thirsty
- slows down your metabolism as well as your body's fat burning process
- increases your blood pressure
- makes you feel fat, bloated, and puffy

I used to use so much salt, I could barely taste the food I was eating. Once I stopped, I started enjoying food so much more. My taste buds came alive. It opened up a whole new world to me. Myriad herbs and spices can be used instead of salt. Experiment with different spices such as pepper, chili powder, and curry.

I challenge you to look at how much salt you are eating and to give up all the unhealthy, salt-laden foods you are used to. Fast food is one of the biggest culprits. It's worth repeating: stop going to fast-food places. Eat natural foods without adding salt. You might want to consider getting rid of your saltshaker altogether.

How Do We Eat?

We've talked about why we eat and what to eat. The next step is learning how to eat.

It's All About Balance

Eating healthy is a balancing act. A proper meal or snack includes the correct balance of protein, carbohydrates, and fats. Your body needs all of them. Many diets on the market today focus on only one of these components of nutrition. That's baloney. You need them all. Protein is the building block for muscle. Carbohydrates give us energy and are our most important source of fuel. Fats will not make us fat, but rather feed our cells and nourish our skin, hair, and nails. All three things are essential to good eating.

My coach, Dr. Rick Katouff, teaches all his clients this formula for balancing macronutrient needs: eat 40-55 percent carbohydrates, 20-30 percent protein, and 20-30 percent fat. This formula helps balance our hormones (serotonin and cortisol). We experience a greater energy level and do not have the highs and lows in blood sugar and insulin levels. This is just one formula. I used it to show you need all three macronutrients in your diet. I want you to focus on having meals and snacks when possible with a balance of good lean protein, complex carbohydrates, and good healthy fats. The ratios can change around a little but the trick is to learn the concept. When you eat this way, you will notice you are less hungry and have more energy throughout the day.

Though we will give you some meal suggestions, you are in charge of planning and preparing most of your meals and snacks for the next ninety days. Try your best to choose your foods based on this formula and the shopping list in appendix B.

Calories Count

The rule of thumb for losing weight is that you need to burn more calories than you take in. Science tells us that one pound of fat is equal to 3500 calories. In order for people to gain or lose a pound, they must increase or decrease their intake of this amount. For example, a daily deficit of 500 calories should result in one pound per week of fat loss. That is the science but because everyone is different, there are some variables to it. I know for me, in the beginning I had no idea how many calories I was actually eating so I had to start writing it down and tracking it. It was a very eye-opening experience. I had been consuming a large amount of calories every day. I lowered my calories to a healthy but sufficient range and added exercise to my plan and I started to lose weight. A healthy example of that would be if you reduced your calories by 300 per day and increased daily activity to burn off an additional 200 calories you would be at your goal of 500 calories burned per day and that should result in a pound a week.

Here are some rules:

Our goal is to burn the fat, not simply starve it. Too many times people decide to "diet" and what they are doing is starving themselves. This is not a healthy or long term approach that is sustainable.

Try to gradually lower your caloric intake. A sudden drop of more than 500 calories can cause your metabolism to slow. Not everyone is the same. This is a process of trial and error. I lowered my calories slowly at first, added exercise, water, sleep, and proper nutrition, eating smaller healthier meals, and my body started to respond by getting rid of the extra fat. Experts agree women should not go below 1200 calories a day and men should not go below 1800. Remember it is "burning" the fat. Your body needs a certain amount of energy to function every day. This process of losing weight may seem complicated, but it really isn't. It is a function of the amount of energy (or calories) a person takes in versus the amount expended.

Word of warning: Beware of crash diets that drastically reduce the type or amount of calories a person takes in. If you were like me and had been consuming too many calories and the wrong type of calories, slowly lower them to a healthy range.

What is a healthy range of calories per day? Referring to the previous chapter, you can figure out what your BMR is and your AMR. Once you know that number, you can determine what you need to do to lose weight. As an example, if your daily calorie needs are 2500 calories, you can consume 2200 calories and try to burn off an additional 200 through exercise. With this formula you can create a deficit of 500 calories in a day. Our goal is sustainable, safe, long-term weight loss.

Each person is different. Some people will lose weight faster than others, so calorie needs for losing weight will fluctuate from person to person. Your goal is to give your body what it needs to survive, thrive, and be healthy while boosting your metabolism and burning excess body fat.

How many calories you consume per day and where you get those calories is a huge part of proper nutrition. Most people have no idea how many calories they eat. This is why we recommend you keep a food journal during the "Challenge." In Part 2 of this book, we include space in the daily challenges to write down what you eat. If you wish, you can buy a small notebook to keep with you at all times to make the process easier for you. However you choose to do it, the important thing is to write down everything you eat and how many calories it has. You can find those numbers on the food label or check out one of my favorite books, *The CalorieKing Calorie, Fat and Carbohydrate Counter* by Allan Borushek, which shows how many calories are in most foods. Plenty of online sources also provide this information. Check out:

- www.thedailyplate.com
- www.calorieking.com
- www.thecaloriecounter.com

I know it may seem like a pain to write everything down, but you have to do it, at least for a few weeks. This is what helped me lose the weight. I needed to see what I was eating and how much so I could track my calorie intake.

Eat, Don't Starve

Many people think that to lose weight, they have to starve themselves. Not true. The best way to eat is four to six small meals a day. Once you figure out how many calories you need to consume to lose weight, you can divvy up that number appropriately throughout the day. Eating small, healthy snacks and meals helps get your metabolism moving, keeps your energy up, keeps your blood sugar stable, and keeps your hunger at bay. It's hard for many folks to eat this way because they forget to eat, and when they finally do, they are starving and end up binging. Don't be one of those people. Set your clock. Put it on your calendar. Do whatever you need to do to eat four to six times a day. Your body will notice the difference.

Tips for Success

Here are our top tips for weight-loss success. Use these tips during the "Challenge" to achieve your health goals and change your food lifestyle for the better.

Portion Control

If you are not a calorie counter, watch your portion sizes. Once your eyes become accustomed to what a normal-sized meal should look like, you will stop overeating. Eating the right portions will help you keep your calorie count under control. This was a big "aha moment" for me. I used to eat mindlessly and way too much. When I switched to eating proper portions that were good for me, I felt great after a meal, not stuffed and ready to pop out of my pants.

Most Americans eat way too much. We have the mentality in this country that bigger is better. We supersize everything, and it is making us fatter. When I was growing up, an 8-ounce soda was the norm. Now it's a 20-ounce or larger, and so many people drink several of those big sodas a day.

One of my favorite books is *The 9-Inch "Diet": Exposing the Big Conspiracy in America* by Alex Bogusky and Chuck Porter. The authors show how our dinner plates have grown from nine inches to twelve inches over the years. We put more food on our plates simply because they are bigger. They also talk about the supersize mentality and explain how so many different foods, such as bagels and sandwiches, have similarly increased in size. When Amy and I discovered this, we went out to a local discount store and bought our family nine-inch plates. Eating off these smaller dishes make us eat a whole lot less.

Try this challenge. Pour yourself a bowl of your favorite cereal in the portion you would normally eat. Now look at the single-serving size on the food label and pour that amount into another bowl (it's usually about one cup of cereal). Notice the difference?

It's likely that you frequently eat three or four servings more than what you are supposed to. It might be time to stop? Let me help you visualize portion sizes. One serving of:

- fruits or vegetables = the size of your fist
- meat, fish, or poultry = the palm of your hand (not counting your fingers)
- dried fruit = a golf ball
- cheese = a dice
- peanut butter = a thumb tip

For more tips on eyeballing the proper portion, check out www.webmd.com/diet/healthtool-portion-size-plate. I also recommend you buy measuring cups for your kitchen so you can correctly measure the proper portion.

Read Labels

Before I buy or eat a food item, I read the label. It shows how many calories are in the food, what the food is made of, and so on. Here is a sample food label:

NUTRITION FACTS

Serving size 1/2 cup (114g)
Servings per container 4

Amount per serving	
Calories 260	Calories from fat 120
	% Daily Value
Total Fat 13g	**20%**
Saturated fat 5g	**25%**
Colesterol 30mg	**10%**
Sodium 660mg	**28%**
Total Carbohydrate 31g	**11%**
Sugars 5g	
Dietary Fiber 0g	
Protein 5g	

Serving Size. The first thing I look for in a food label is the serving size. When I pick up two products I am comparing, I want to make sure the serving size is listed the same. Next I look at how many servings there are per container. Remember, it's all about portion control. For example, if I do not know that a package contains two servings, I will be ingesting double the calories listed on the label if I eat the whole package.

Calories. I always pay attention to the number of calories per serving. In general, a food with:

- 40 calories per serving is low in calories
- 100 calories per serving is moderate in calories
- 400 calories or more per serving is high in calories

Fats. I avoid foods with trans fats and choose foods with less than 5 grams of fat per serving. Also, make note of the number of calories from fat. Avoid foods with fat calories that exceed 20 to 25 percent of the total calories (divide the number of calories from fat by the total number of calories to find the percentage).

Sodium. I choose only foods that are low in sodium since I want to keep my daily sodium intake under 2300 milligrams.

Sugar. The sugar content also should be low. I read labels and avoid eating anything with added sugar in it.

Fiber. Remember, you need to have anywhere from 25-30 grams of fiber per day, so try to choose foods that have at least 3 grams of fiber per serving.

When it comes to ingredients, I have a simple rule. If I cannot pronounce it or there are a lot on the list, I won't eat it. My oldest son wanted some cheese crackers one day. I told him he could have them if he read to me all the ingredients on the side of the box. He got halfway through and quit. "Dad," he sighed, "I don't want them anymore." Just stick with natural and whole foods as much as possible and you'll be okay.

The Trade Game

Amy and I live in South Carolina, and we like to say that in the South, people can take a healthy food and make it unhealthy. Ever hear of fried okra? The okra part is great, but the fried part? Not so much. It's time to understand that you can substitute healthy and delicious meals for the junk you have been eating.

There is a misconception that eating healthy means sacrificing taste. People also often think they have to give up everything when they diet. When I began my fitness journey, I was taught to think differently. I had to remind myself that I did not have to give up taste and that there were many food choices out there. It was possible to replace the old things I used to eat with new things that were just as yummy. I can't begin to tell you how changing this thought process helped me.

I walked into a farmer's market one day and had an epiphany. I saw a whole bunch of vibrantly colored and delicious looking fruits and vegetables that I had never eaten before. I mean, I saw five different varieties of apples, all of which had a distinct taste. This helped me reprogram my brain from focusing on the fried, sweet, and processed foods I used to enjoy to focusing on the bigger picture that I was gaining health.

Substitution is the name of the game. Chef Devin Alexander has published many great cookbooks (my personal favorite is *The Most Decadent Diet Ever: The cookbook that reveals the secrets to cooking your favorites in a healthier way*) where she takes comfort food recipes, such as eggplant parmesan, popcorn chicken, and pasta dishes, and provides healthy recipe alternatives that taste just as good. You can buy her cookbooks and start cooking some delectable meals.

Break out of your comfort zone. Look at what you are eating and ask yourself if there is a healthier ingredient. Check out my suggestions below. Let these guide you in making the right food choices.

Instead of This:	**Try This:**
mayonnaise	mustard
ketchup	salsa
ice cream	frozen yogurt
white rice	brown rice
regular pasta	wheat or quinoa pasta
white bread	wheat bread or wraps or Ezekiel bread
ground beef	ground turkey or chicken
whole milk	skim milk
sour cream	plain low-fat yogurt
white, creamy sauces (e.g., Alfredo)	red, tomato sauces (marinara)
salt	herb seasonings (pepper, Mrs. Dash)

Eating on the Run

I know it can be hard to make healthy food choices when you're away from home, but it is doable. You want to always think ahead. If you know you will be traveling, carry healthy snacks and meals with you. Cut up some fruit or veggies and stick them in baggies to munch on. If you can make a healthy salad or sandwich to pack, do that too.

I know sometimes you have no choice but to eat at a fast-food place, deli, convenience store, or restaurant. When you have to grab food on the go, stick with natural foods. Most places sell fruit and packaged salads (just use fat-free dressings or oil and vinegar). Your choices may be limited, but you will always find a healthy option somewhere.

If you are at a restaurant, stick with grilled proteins such as chicken breast or fish, salads with oil and vinegar dressing on the side, and vegetable sides. Stay away from cheesy or fried foods and bread. Always skip the bread. If you can, plan ahead. If you know you are going out to eat somewhere, check online for a menu before you get there. Many online menus include nutritional information. Check out your options and choose your meal beforehand. Also, many places have "healthy options" on their menu. And when in doubt, ask your waiter for meal recommendations.

Getting Started

We've talked about why we eat, what to eat, how to eat, and have given you some great tips. Now it's time for some action.

Step 1: Time to Take Out the Trash

The first thing you need to do is to get rid of all the junk and processed foods in your house. I'm serious. I was so addicted to sugar and junk food that I needed to get radical. If you don't get radical in the beginning, you may not be as successful. You will still be fighting those cravings, and it will sabotage your ability to lose weight.

I found out that, much like any other addiction, our bodies have a chemical reaction to sweets and sugar, so there will be a period of cravings and adjustment. I choose not to keep those foods in the house because when I am tempted to snack, I do not want those foods around. Moderation is a skill you can learn once you've lost the weight. Now is the time to get serious. (If you feel guilty about throwing food away, donate it to a local food pantry or shelter.)

You may have to get rid of more food than you keep. Open your fridge and get into your pantry and immediately get rid of:

- Anything that is processed and fake, including processed lunch meats, soda, margarine, processed cheese, white rice, white pasta, white breads, instant foods (canned soups, macaroni and cheese, boxed meals), sweets (cookies, cakes, ice cream), and snacks (crackers and chips)
- Anything that has a long shelf life
- Anything that has refined or high fructose sugar or has ingredients that you cannot pronounce
- Anything that is not natural or minimally processed

Step 2: Time to Go Shopping

After your purge, plan today to go grocery shopping for foods that are good for you. Here is a list of what Amy and I consider our food staples, and we always keep plenty around to whip up meals and snacks. You can also pull from the comprehensive shopping list in appendix B.

- Old-fashioned oatmeal. Use this instead of the instant varieties. Oatmeal is easy to make and one of the best foods you can eat in the morning. It's packed with fiber, and you can mix it with honey, cinnamon, fruit, flaxseed, or nuts.
- Canned beans (pinto, red, chickpeas, kidney, black, take your pick). Beans are low in fat and high in fiber, calcium, and iron.
- Fresh and frozen vegetables. They are easy to make steamed or cooked in a little bit of extra virgin olive oil. We especially love spinach.
- Fresh fruit. We always have fresh fruit available because it's the perfect snack. It's prepackaged by God in a perfect size.
- Brown rice. We love the kind that you boil in a bag. We mix our rice with salsa and hummus and vegetables. It is filling and delicious.
- Mustard and salsa. These are two great condiments we always use. I love fresh salsa and make it myself when I can. I switched from mayo to mustard and have never looked back.
- Tuna. If I'm in a hurry, I can put a package of tuna in my lunch sack and head out the door. I mix it with mustard, olive oil, and chickpeas when I put it in a salad. It has tons of protein.
- Eggs. We always have eggs around. They have been described as the perfect food. They are great scrambled or boiled and chopped up into salads.
- Hummus. We make our own hummus, but it's just as easy to buy premade hummus, especially when you are just getting started. It's great to use as a spread or in a dip.
- Lean protein such as chicken, turkey, and fish. Buy frozen or put fresh in your freezer if you don't plan to use it right away.
- Olive oil. This is the best kind for cooking and sautéing.

Other Tools We Love

There are other items that you'll want to have on hand to help you with better nutrition. Use these tools to make your weight-loss journey easier. You don't have to run out and get these all at once. But eventually, for a permanent lifestyle change, they will help you keep track of what you eat and will make your life in the kitchen a lot easier.

Calorie counter guide. You know how important it is to know how many calories you are putting into your body. We keep recommending *The CalorieKing Calorie, Fat and Carb Counter* book for a reason.

Kitchen scales and measuring cups. What great tools for portion control. When a recipe calls for four ounces of chicken or a cup of strawberries, these items will ensure you get the right amount.

Mini food processor. This small kitchen appliance costs around twenty dollars and comes in handy for so many different things. You can save money by using it to make your own salsa, guacamole, hummus, dressings, and other things. Ours is constantly in use.

Pan with a large steamer basket. This is a valuable tool to steam large amounts of vegetables. We put in all of our veggies that we want to steam at one time and divide them up after they are cooked. It saves so much time.

There is just so much information out there on eating healthy. A number of great resources have helped us on our journey and made us more knowledgeable. We shared some of them with you already, but here are a few more:

- *Winning by Losing: Drop the Weight, Change Your Life* by Jillian Michaels
- *Are You Ready! Take Charge, Lose Weight, Get in Shape, and Change Your Life Forever* by Bob Harper
- *The Eat-Clean Diet: Fast Fat-Loss that Lasts Forever* by Tosca Reno
- *Let's Do Lunch: Eating All the Calories and Carbs You Want to Lose Weight* by Roger Troy Wilson
- *Fast Food Nation* by Eric Schlosser
- *The Biggest Loser* cookbooks
- *Your Body's Many Cries for Water: You Are Not Sick, You Are Thirsty* by F. Batmanghelidj

Meal Plans

In appendix C, we provide you a seven-day eating plan that includes breakfast, lunch, dinner, and two snack options. I did not include portions because you should determine your own portions based on your caloric threshold. For example, Amy stayed around 1200 calories most of the time, so she would have five ounces of chicken whereas I would have eight ounces because I was at a higher caloric intake.

We are not dieticians. These meals and snacks are based on what our nutritionists suggested that we eat and what we know works for us. Feel free to get some healthy cookbooks to use in creating your own daily menus. We've included some of our favorite recipes for you in appendix D.

Since you will be planning most of your meals and snacks, remember the guidelines we taught you above and especially the three keys to determining what you will eat every day:

- Choose meals and snacks that are within your daily calorie needs for losing weight.
- Make sure 90 percent of your food choices are whole, fresh, and natural (fruits, veggies, lean meats, and whole grains).
- Eat the right balance of protein, carbs, and fats.

I hope you are getting excited. While knowing how and what to eat is a critical element in weight loss, exercise is just as important. It's time to start learning why and how to get your body moving.

4

Activate Your Body

A Note from Phil

I want you to enjoy the fullest life you can. I know you are on the right path because you are already reading this book. You are dreaming again of the desires that you want in your life. You have recognized where you are physically and have set some goals of what you want to accomplish in the next ninety days. You have learned what foods you need to eat to fuel your body and how many calories you need to lose weight.

Today you will learn about the fourth key in our DREAM principle—*activate your body*. Here's the deal. If you want to lose weight, cutting back on calories is simply not enough. Exercise needs to be a regular part of your lifestyle to help you get to and maintain a healthy weight.

Before I got started on my weight-loss journey, I shuddered at the thought of exercise. In my mind, fitness training was something other people did. I never fully saw the value in it. But since being on *The Biggest Loser* and maintaining a healthy lifestyle, I have seen the amazing benefits of keeping fit. Not only does fitness improve your body, but it does wonders for your mental and emotional well-being.

When I was on the show, I would have mini panic attacks before our trainers worked out with us. Exercise scared the living daylights out of me. I soon realized I was dealing with a deeper issue. Secretly, I had always wanted to be athletic, but I never was. As a kid, I played sports with my friends at my church. When I was in the eighth grade, I tried out for basketball but didn't make the team. When I got to high school, I played some tennis and golf, but something about the failure with basketball stuck in my mind.

When I was eighteen, I decided to join a local gym. I was determined to get into good shape. I met with a personal trainer who worked me out so hard, when the session was over, I crawled to the bathroom and threw up. Though I had paid for my membership, I never went back. Once again, I felt like a failure.

It took being on the show to face my fears of failing when it came to fitness.

While struggling through grueling workouts, I had no choice but to endure the process and face my fears. I slowly came to realize that I had to change my attitude toward exercise. My past defeats did not have to dictate my future health. I wanted to be healthy. I wanted my family to be healthy. And I had to work through my mental block to make those things happen.

The Benefits of Exercise

Here are several awesome benefits that come with regular exercise:

- You'll lose weight. Cardiovascular (or aerobic) exercise is what is going to help you burn fat and make the pounds peel off.
- Weight training will help shape your body. Building your muscle will give you the tight and toned body you always wanted.
- For every pound of muscle you gain, you burn calories, even when you are sleeping.
- The more you exercise, the more your metabolism will increase. This also helps your body burn more calories.
- Exercise boosts your immune system, helping you fight off sickness and even serious health problems such as diabetes and heart disease. It also reduces high blood pressure.
- Exercise reduces stress. This is my favorite. When you exercise, various brain chemicals are released that make you feel relaxed. I feel so much better when I work out than if I don't. Even something as simple as walking will help to clear your mind and put you in a more positive mindset.
- Exercise does wonders for your cardiovascular system. It helps keep the blood circulating through your heart and lungs, and when your heart and lungs work more efficiently, you have more energy.
- Exercise improves your sleep. Getting enough sleep, about seven to eight hours a night, is important to good health. Research has shown that exercising helps you sleep better.

What Is Exercise?

What do you think about when you hear the word *exercise*? What thoughts or pictures form in your mind? Maybe you have visions of scary equipment you don't think you can ever figure out how to use. Maybe you feel overwhelmed at the thought of following a workout plan that seems way too complicated to do a couple times a week. Maybe the thought of exercising frustrates you because you don't think you have the best balance or coordination.

Whatever your reasons for not working out, by now I hope you understand that you must just do it. From now on, exercise is going to become a permanent fixture in your life. I want you to get excited about it. I'm here to help you through this process, to lessen whatever fears you have, and to help you realize that exercise can be fun and creative.

So what is exercise? The bottom line is that all activity counts. If your body is moving around doing something, that's a good thing. It means you are burning calories. Think about it like this. You burn more calories standing than you do sitting. You burn more calories walking than you do standing. You burn more calories running than walking. You get the idea.

Let's start by talking about the traditional ways of exercising that you have probably already heard about. It's important to understand the basics because even if you hire a personal trainer, he or she going to give you the same fundamentals.

Cardiovascular Training

Cardiovascular training might conjure up images of people jumping around and sweating like crazy. Well, you're on the right track. Cardio is the key to fat loss. On average, you can burn about five hundred calories in a one-hour cardio session. This helps create the calorie deficit you need to lose weight. If you forget everything else, just remember cardio is what will ignite your weight loss. On the ranch, we were on the treadmill, the stepper, the elliptical machine, and other cardio machines for hours. And I literally mean hours. You don't have to spend that much time doing cardio, of course. I just want you to see the direct link between this exercise and fat loss.

To put it simply, cardio exercise raises your heart rate. You are working out at the right intensity at the beginning of this challenge if you are slightly out of breath but can still hold a conversation. How long should you do a cardio session? I recommend you start out doing thirty minutes three times a week and work your way up to forty-five to sixty-minute sessions five times a week.

Here are some examples of ways to get your cardio in. I'm giving you a wide variety to work with depending on whether you are a member of a gym. While you don't have to join a gym right now, it might help you stay motivated. It's your choice.

If you have equipment or go to a gym with cardio equipment, you can use the:

- Treadmill
- Elliptical machine
- Stair climber
- Stationary bike
- Rowing machine
- Pool for lap swimming

If you join a gym, you can also take the cardio classes they offer such as:

- Kickboxing
- Cardio Blast
- Spin
- Water aerobics
- Step classes
- Zumba

If you play tennis, soccer, or basketball, you can get your cardio in that way. You might want to join a local community team or even create your own sports team. If you don't belong to a gym, no worries. You can:

- Rollerblade
- Walk or run in your neighborhood or around a local high school track
- Dance inside your house with high-energy music (have your kids join you)
- Hike a trail at a local park
- Rent a cardio DVD from the library and do it in your living room
- Find an early morning exercise program on TV and join in with the trainer
- Go to the local high school and walk up and down the bleachers
- Take your dog for a brisk walk
- Rake leaves
- Do heavy housework, such as mopping floors and vacuuming
- Play outdoor games such as Frisbee or catch with your kids

Whatever you choose to do, just make sure you get and keep your heart rate up for at least thirty to forty-five minutes.

Weight and Resistance Training

The other piece to getting fit is weight and resistance training. This can sound intimidating if all you think about are the big and bulky guys grunting at the gym. But it's not all about the meatheads. The reason a lot of *The Biggest Loser* competitors looked so shapely and had minimal loose skin after they lost so much weight is that they strength trained. With cardio you will lose weight, but your body will still be the same shape, only smaller. True body transformation with strong muscles that make you look tight and toned comes from strength training. Once you start lifting weights, you will see your body shape changing and your weight being better redistributed in just three months.

How do you strength train? So much information is out there on how to weight train, such as doing slow sets, supersets, high reps with low weight, low reps with high weights, and so on. We will stick with the basics for these next three months so you don't get overwhelmed. In appendix E, you will find a three-tier workout plan for the next ninety days, which includes strength training exercises you can do at home.

But Phil, I Just Don't Have Time to Exercise

Many people complain they have no time to exercise. You might think I'm crazy for asking you to find thirty minutes or an hour almost every day out of the next ninety days to focus on fitness. You might think it's an impossible task to commit to. Here's something to think about—you don't have to exercise all at one time. You can break it up into spurts. If you exercise an hour at a time or for fifteen minutes four times a day, you will still get the same benefits.

See how manageable that sounds? I know all of you can sneak in fifteen minutes of exercise here and there throughout your day. I have a friend who has two jobs; he is both a school teacher and a personal trainer. You can imagine how busy he is, but he always gets mini workouts in throughout the day. Some days he'll do 30 pushups every hour between classes. That's 240 pushups a day. Incredible.

I know you may not be able to "drop down and give me 30" every hour, but there is always a way to be active even if your schedule is jam-packed. And let's face it folks, if you want to change your life and lose weight, you are going to have to make time. No excuses.

How Hard Do I Need to Exercise?

I've said before that exercise is activity that gets your heart rate up. If you are breathing harder and your heart is beating faster than it would if you were sitting down, you are exercising.

If you are working at a *moderate-intensity* level, you are sweating and able to carry on a conversation, but not able to belt out a favorite song. Walking, water aerobics, and riding a bike on a flat surface are examples of moderate-intensity activities.

Once your body adapts to a workout routine, you are going to want to make your workouts more intense. At a *high-intensity* level, you'll be able to say only a few words without pausing to breathe. Some examples of high-intensity activity include running, playing basketball or soccer, and walking on an incline.

One great way to gauge the intensity of your exercise is by measuring your heart rate as you work out. You can do this either manually by taking your pulse on the inside of your wrist or you can wear a heart rate monitor.

Your maximum heart rate is when you are exercising at the highest level of intensity. This number is determined by subtracting your age from 220. I obviously don't expect you to start out exercising for an hour at your maximum heart rate, but I do want your workouts to increase your heart rate to between 50-85 percent of your maximum rate. This is your "target heart rate zone." The following chart lists the target heart rate zones and maximum heart rates based on your age.

AGE	Target HR Zone 50–85% of max.	Average Maximum Heart Rate 100%
20 years	100–170 beats per minute	200 beats per minute
25 years	98–166 beats per minute	195 beats per minute
30 years	95–162 beats per minute	190 beats per minute
35 years	93–157 beats per minute	185 beats per minute
40 years	90–153 beats per minute	180 beats per minute
45 years	88–149 beats per minute	175 beats per minute
50 years	85–145 beats per minute	170 beats per minute
55 years	83–140 beats per minute	165 beats per minute
60 years	80–136 beats per minute	160 beats per minute
65 years	78–132 beats per minute	155 beats per minute
70 years	75–128 beats per minute	150 beats per minute

These guidelines can help you gauge the intensity of your workouts, but I don't want you to get too bogged down by these numbers. Remember, the most important thing is to move. A good start is just to get off the couch and walk around the block.

Variety Is the Spice of...Exercise

Another important thing to remember as you start working out is to include some variation. You don't want to do the same thing every day because your body will get used to your routine. Let's say you start out walking around your neighborhood every day for an hour. Great. You notice you are feeling better and are beginning to lose weight. After you do this for two or three weeks, suddenly your weight loss slows down even though you are doing the same thing. You wonder what on earth is happening. Your body is simply getting used to the activity. It has figured out your routine, and the growth you once experienced from walking has stopped.

Amy and I are always switching up our workouts. We don't do the same thing every day. Some days we run. Some days we swim. Some days we take a weight-training class at the gym. This helps our body to be constantly surprised so we are always gaining the benefits of exercise.

Another way of varying your workouts is to vary the intensity with interval training. Training this way gives your metabolism a shock to its system. Interval training is getting your heart rate really high for a short amount of time (fifteen seconds to one minute), and bringing it back down for a few more minutes, and then repeating the process. This is not hard to do. If you start out walking, add some spurts of brisk walking to your routine. If you walk on a treadmill, every few minutes hit the grade button and increase your incline for thirty seconds.

If you are a member of a gym, you can mix up your routine by taking classes that include aerobic activity and weight training. Check out the schedule at your local gym and see what they have.

Tips and Resources

As you get started on your fitness journey, here are a few recommendations. You don't need to do all of them right now, but keep them in mind as you incorporate exercise into your new, healthy lifestyle.

Get a good pair of running shoes. I recommend getting these as soon as possible. Go to an athletic store and get fitted for the right athletic shoe for your feet. We all can't wear the same kind of sneaker. Each person has a different arch and instep and different fitness goals. Spend some time with a professional in the store and talk about these things. He or she will suggest the right shoe for your needs.

Buy a water bottle. This is a necessity right off the bat. You must have a water bottle with you at all times. By now you know you need to be drinking water all the time. Buy a water bottle that holds at least twenty ounces and that will keep your water cool.

Get some workout clothes. You don't have to go nuts and spend tons of money. If this is not in your budget right now, don't worry. Just wear some oversized T-shirts and shorts you have in the house. When you are ready to buy (since the clothes you're now wearing will soon become very baggy), buy clothes that are comfortable and reasonably priced based on your budget.

I suggest investing in clothes made from moisture-wicking material, especially if you cycle or run. You can ask the clothing specialist at a store for help picking out the right apparel. Most people wear clothes made of cotton when they work out, but cotton absorbs sweat and clings to your skin. Moisture-wicking apparel gets rids of moisture quickly and keeps you drier.

If you are a woman, buy a few good sports bras that will give you support and keep you comfortable.

Another great investment is a pair of compression shorts you can wear underneath your regular shorts or workout pants. They help with the chaffing that comes when your thighs rub together.

Buy a heart rate monitor. While this is not a must, it is a great tool for judging the intensity of your workouts and how many calories you are burning.

To gym or not to gym? You do not have to join a gym, but there are many advantages to being a member—trainers who can help you on your way, different classes and activities so you can try new things and switch up your workouts, and people you meet who may eventually become your workout buddies. This has happened to both Amy and me. We have met some of our closest friends at our local gym.

I know it might be intimidating at first to work out in front of others. This is a fear you might have to work through. Try not to think about what others are thinking about you. Who cares what they think. You are there to focus on your health goals. You are there to feel and look better. You are there to ultimately gain a better life. Don't let your insecurities keep you from joining a gym.

Most gyms offer free passes. Try out a couple of facilities in your area and choose the one you like best. Pick a place that motivates you and moves you forward and offers a comfortable and positive environment that you can grow in.

Fitness equipment for your home. If you are not going to join a gym and you want to keep some equipment in your home, this is what we recommend. Our workout plans (see appendix E) list exercises you can do with some of these items. Otherwise, take a look at the many instructional fitness DVDs out there, find one you like, and buy the required equipment to do those workouts. Some basic (and inexpensive) home equipment includes:

- Jump rope
- Dumbbells (3 lbs–25 lbs)
- Yoga mat
- Workout and instructional DVDs
- Medicine ball
- Inflatable large ball
- Resistance bands

The Plan

The 90-Day Fitness Challenge comes with three fitness plans, one plan for each month. You'll find these plans in appendix E at the back of the book. The first is an easy one to get you started and get you comfortable with the basics. Since you are probably a beginner at exercise, it will include activities tailored for someone just starting out on a weight-loss journey. The plan for the second month is more challenging and will encourage you to try different exercises. The third plan is the most intense with heavier weight workouts and higher-intensity cardio. It will also help your fitness level grow and help you to stay motivated.

Don't feel the need to attach yourself to all of our recommendations. They are meant to guide you on your way, but you should commit to a plan that you enjoy and that works for you. If you want to get a personal trainer, by all means go for it. You can even tailor your routine on your own. There are great resources out there to help you get started. We like:

- *Shape Magazine's Ultimate Body Book: 4 Weeks to Your Best Abs, Butt, Thighs, and More* by Linda Shelton with Angela Hynes
- *Fitness for Dummies* by Suzanne Schlosberg and Liz Neporent

- *8 Minutes in the Morning for Extra-Easy Weight Loss* by Jorge Cruise
- *The 10-Minute Total Body Breakthrough* by Sean Foy, Nellie Sabin, Mike Smolinski, and William Sears, MD
- *The Biggest Loser Fitness Program: Fast, Safe, and Effective Workouts to Target and Tone Your Trouble Spots—Adapted from NBC's Hit Show!* by *The Biggest Loser* experts and cast, with Maggie Greenwood-Robinson

When you get to the daily challenges in Part 2 of this book, you will see each day has space to record your workouts. Write down what you do every day. You might want a separate notebook to do this. The key is to monitor your fitness levels and see where you are increasing your intensity and weights.

Remember, being active is a key part of living a healthy lifestyle. Gaining health and losing weight means getting off that couch and moving around. You'll quickly notice the difference in how you feel once you substitute an active lifestyle for a sedentary one.

Losing weight brings tremendous positive life changes. For us, one of the big things we learned was our responsibility to help others better their lives. When we saw how drastic our lives changed by taking care of our bodies, we knew we had to pass the message along. You'll see what we mean in the next chapter when we explore our final key in the DREAM principle.

5

Make a Difference in the Lives of Others

A Word from Amy

The final key in the DREAM principle is to *make a difference in the lives of others*. I believe this is the fundamental step of the entire principle. When we consciously look for ways to give of ourselves and our resources, we open ourselves to a wonderful world of possibilities. We are planting seeds that can sprout up in millions of wonderful ways.

When Phil and I were given the opportunity to go on *The Biggest Loser*, we knew it was a direct blessing from God. We felt His presence and grace the entire time we were there. We had an overwhelming feeling that just being there was a vehicle that the Lord was going to use to fulfill His plan; we were just along for the ride.

And what a wild ride it has been! How could we have known that literally millions of people would watch us and be influenced by our story? How could we have known that we would be able to travel around the country and share what we have learned and see lives changed as a result? How could we have known that we would be able to write this book that you are now reading that we hope will better your life? How could we have known that the true prize of being on the show was knowing that we had made a difference in other people's lives?

My husband and I didn't have a clue what was in store for us. But God did.

Jesus says in Luke 6:38, "Give, and you will receive. Your gift will return to you in full—pressed down, shaken together to make room for more, running over, and poured into your lap. The amount you give will determine the amount you get back." Giving is a spiritual law. If we give, we will receive. The second part of that verse shows us that the amount that we give will determine the amount given to us. I like to look at it this way. If we use a teaspoon, then we will get a teaspoon back. If we use a dump truck, then we will get a dump truck load of blessing back. It's simple. The more we give, the more we get back.

It's so easy in this fast-paced world to get caught up in ourselves. After all, we have so many responsibilities to tend to. We work, have families, are involved in our churches and communities, and have to take care of our health. Sometimes it seems as if there are not enough hours in the day to do everything we need to do for ourselves, let alone help others. This is often why we fail to make a difference. We don't have time. We're just too busy.

But you know what? Excuses like those don't cut it.

Throughout this fitness challenge over the next ninety days, you will continue to learn how to become more healthy and in control of your body. Just as an infant slowly crawls and then learns to walk and eventually run, we believe that you will undergo a similar metamorphosis. As you begin to change your health for the better, you can make a difference by remembering those who are similarly trapped in their bodies. Help them learn to run. Pay the gift of health forward. Tell others about the "Challenge" and encourage them through the process.

Giving Brings Joy, Gratitude, and Blessings

Helping others is essential for experiencing joy. When we make it a practice to acknowledge our God-given gifts and look for ways to share them with others, it is only natural to be thankful for all we have. When we focus on filling the needs of others, we are less likely to focus on the negative aspects of our lives.

When I was younger, I volunteered for a community organization that made and delivered food baskets to needy families during Christmas. I had lived a fairly comfortable life growing up, although I viewed myself as poor when I compared what I had to what my friends had. In hindsight, I never lacked for anything. There was always food on the table and clothes on my back. But all I saw then was what I didn't have.

My perspective of poverty completely changed the day I delivered gift baskets to those families. I remember one family in particular. I walked through their front door and was shocked at how dilapidated their home was. There were holes in the floor so large you could see the dirt underneath the house. In one corner I saw three children huddled around a black-and-white television that barely got reception. They were covered with dirt and grime and looked so sad. The father was in bed, too sick to get up. The mother, a gracious lady, told us that because her husband was ill, he was out of work; she had to stay home with the children, so they had no income. It broke my heart.

I'll never forget how excited this woman and her kids were to see our gifts. It made my heart so happy that even though I couldn't change their situation,

I could do a little something to bring joy to their day. Suddenly, the problems I had seemed a million miles away. My troubles were nothing compared to this family's desperate situation. I saw my life in a completely different light and had a better attitude of appreciating all I had.

When you make a difference in others, your life changes.

A friend who is a real estate agent recently had a difficult year in sales compared to previous years. He was constantly worried, depressed, and always focused on how bad things were. One day he told me that he had been asked to help serve food once a week to a group of homeless people. He had never done anything like that before, but thought it would be a great thing to do. He told me that once he started serving in that way, he noticed his real estate business started picking up. The month that he got involved in that ministry, he wrote sixteen real estate contracts. Previously, it had taken him a year to get that much business.

My friend gave to those who had no home of their own, and the windows of heaven opened for him to sell people homes. What a sense of humor God has!

There are so many ways to give to others. You could give money, your time, your knowledge, your talents. You can volunteer at a local shelter. You can sponsor a child in a refugee camp. You can help a neighborhood child learn to read. You can offer to carry groceries for an elderly person. Your options are endless.

Just think about your own life and what you have to offer. Identify the gifts you have inside of you. Are you a loyal friend, an eloquent speaker, a fabulous cook, a great gardener, a nurturing mother, or a talented musician? Whatever the gift God has given you, find a way to use it to bless others. I promise you that your life will change.

The Gift of Words

One of the easiest ways to give to others is by encouraging them. It's simple to do, doesn't take much time, and makes a world of difference. It's a wonder why we don't do it all the time. How many people do you know who could use a word of encouragement? I'm sure there are many.

A friend of mine likes to send out daily text messages of encouragement to the folks on his contacts list. One day a businessman that he knew only casually called him up and asked him out for coffee. They had a great time chatting. Right before they were getting up to leave, the businessman said to my friend, "I wanted to tell you that you saved my life." My friend had no idea what the man was talking about. I mean, he barely knew the guy. The man explained that he had gone through a terrible year financially. He was in the construction supply business, and when the economy took a turn for the worse, he was left with $800,000 of unpaid invoices that he knew would probably never get paid to him.

One day he needed to make payroll, and he didn't have any money to do it or even to pay his personal bills. The man looked over toward the fax machine and saw his pistol lying on the shelf above it. He truly believed that taking his life was the only way out. He moved his chair to reach for the gun, and just as he did, his phone beeped with a text message. He glanced at the screen and stopped cold as he read the simple message my friend had sent—"Trust in the Lord." These words brought him instant comfort. He knew that God had used my friend to send him that message at exactly the right moment.

You never know how you might make a difference in someone else's life. All my friend did was use his gift of encouragement, and look what happened.

There are all kinds of gifts inside of you. God has placed them there for a purpose. You may have let them lie dormant, but they are there whether you let them out or not. The Bible says that the gifts and callings of God are "irrevocable" (Romans 11:29). That means that once God gives you a gift or a calling, you can't get rid of it. It is forever a part of you. It is designed to be used to make an impact on the world and the people in it.

So use it!

Remembering the Blessings

When I look back on my life, I always remember the times when people gave me something just because they wanted to bless me. They didn't give because they wanted something in return or because they wanted a pat on the back. They gave because they wanted to make my life better.

When I was pregnant with my oldest son, Austin, Phil and I were living in Puyallup, Washington, a little town near Seattle. We had lived there only a short time, and I was three thousand miles from any family. We didn't have much money, and a part of me was a little uncertain about how we were going to take care of this baby. I was also a little down because I knew that a baby shower was out of the question since we were so new to town. We had just started going to a local church and had barely begun to make a few friends. One Sunday afternoon, much to my surprise, the ladies of the church threw me a baby shower. There were people I didn't even know who showed up to give me gifts and wish me well. I felt the most amazing outpouring of love that day.

Another instance that comes to mind is when Phil and I celebrated one of our early Christmases as newlyweds. We lived in a sketchy neighborhood in a tiny house that had no heat. Phil and I put a space heater in our bedroom at night. When we had to bathe, we would run to the bathroom, turn on the hot water, and then run back to the warm bedroom. When the tub was full, we would run back to the bathroom, jump in the tub, bathe, and run back to the warm bedroom again to get dressed. We did this all winter that year.

This particular Christmas Eve I came home to that little rundown house to find a huge platter of homemade cookies and Christmas candy on our front doorstep. A family in our church had a tradition of baking together the week before Christmas, and on Christmas Eve they would go to specially chosen homes and, like little elves, deliver their goodies. The fact that they spent their time to make this special gift for us deeply touched our hearts. When our children were old enough, Phil and I decided to adopt that Christmas tradition as our own. Our boys love to do it because it makes them feel good to give to others and especially to see the smiles on the faces of those we serve.

When we remember how we have been incredibly blessed, we have a responsibility to pay it forward and give to others. I hope my children do the same thing with their children and give back for the many times they have received.

When God Moves You to Make a Difference

Have you ever had a feeling that you should call someone to see how they are doing or pop by and visit them, only to find out that they are going through a difficult time and could use your help? I believe those are the moments that God is directing you to use your gifts. If we are sensitive to these feelings, we will find that we are able to affect so many lives in ways we never imagined.

On the morning of the casting call for *The Biggest Loser*, I was irritated at Phil because he was moving way too slow for me. I wanted to hurry up and get to the auditions so we could be one of the first ones in line. When we drove up to the building, he let me out while he went to park the car. I stood in line and started venting to the first person that looked nice enough to listen to me blow off some steam. That person was Rae, and she said that she had wanted to get in line early as well, but one thing led to another and she and her best friend, Lolo, got there at the same time we did.

Open casting calls require you to stand in line for hours while you wait for a casting director to see you. As you can imagine, you get to know a lot about the people standing in line with you. Phil and I chatted with Rae and Lolo for hours. By the end of the day, the four of us were laughing hysterically, and by the time we got to the casting director, we had caused such a scene that he had no choice but to give all four of us a callback to the next round.

We went out to lunch to celebrate and exchanged phone numbers and email addresses before we went our separate ways. As it turned out, Phil and I made the show; Rae and Lolo, unfortunately, did not. Still, we remained in close contact with them. Lolo visited us several times at our home in South Carolina, and eventually we invited her to live with us and help us with our kids when we traveled. To our excitement, she said yes. Lolo has been a part of our family ever since.

The story doesn't stop there. Since she has been living with us, Lolo has lost seventy pounds. She says that it wasn't God's plan for her to go to the ranch because He brought the ranch to her. Who knows what would have happened if we had gotten to the casting call as early as I wanted to. Maybe we wouldn't have met Rae and Lolo. Maybe we wouldn't have gotten a callback. We definitely wouldn't have Lolo in our lives now. God had a hand in timing our meeting just right so that we would all be there together and eventually make a huge impact on each other's lives.

Be sensitive to what God is prompting you to do and be open to what is going on around you. Don't be like I once was, so caught up in plans and schedules that you miss the bigger picture and don't realize that God may have a plan for you that you don't know about. Endeavour to be led by His voice.

You are made by God to live an abundant life. When God made the world, He said it was good. Then He created man to enjoy His creation and to rule and take care of it. Many of us have let life be in charge of us instead of God's plan of abundance. Now is the time to reverse that pattern.

I love what the author of the Book of Hebrews wrote, "Therefore, since we are surrounded by such a huge crowd of witnesses to the life of faith, let us strip off every weight that slows us down, especially the sin that so easily trips us up. And let us run with endurance the race God has set before us. We do this by keeping our eyes on Jesus, the champion who initiates and perfects our faith" (Hebrews 12:1-2).

When I read these verses, I visualize the grandstands of heaven cheering us on in our spiritual race and in our lives. Think of loved ones that have gone on before you. I believe they are in that "huge crowd of witnesses." I believe they are watching you and are waiting with anticipation to see if you will conquer the challenges or be complacent and let circumstances take you over.

This challenge is about more than just your body. It's about changing on the inside and watching the results on the outside. It's about knowing that you are strong and powerful and can do all things through Christ. And it is especially about passing on wisdom and serving and helping others so they, too, can finish the race.

As you venture into the next ninety days, live each day to better yourself so that you can make a difference in this world. I know you can do it!

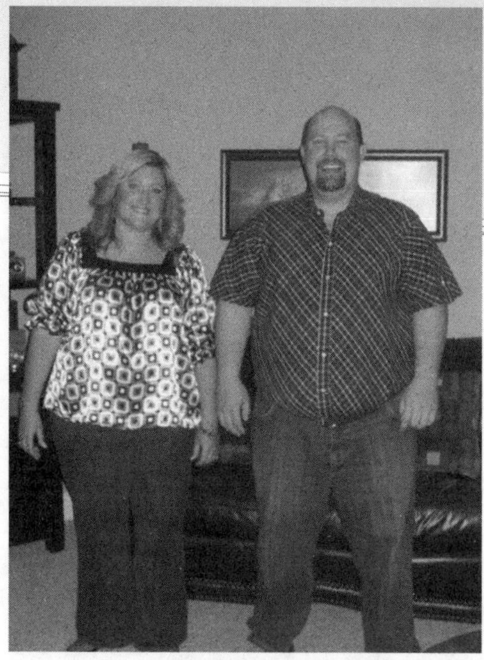

Phil and Amy, May 2008, before their transformation

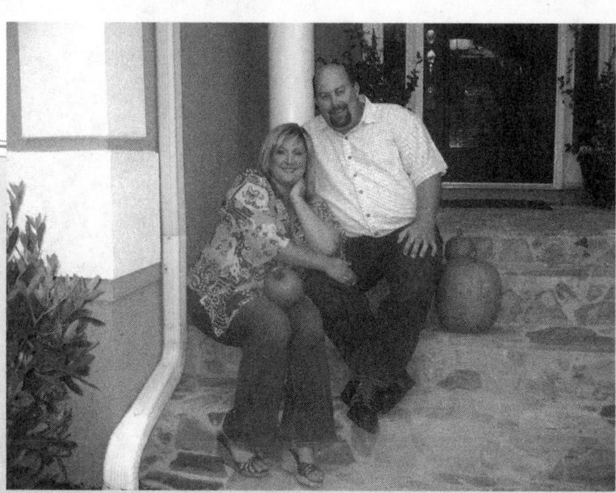

Phil and Amy, Fall 2007

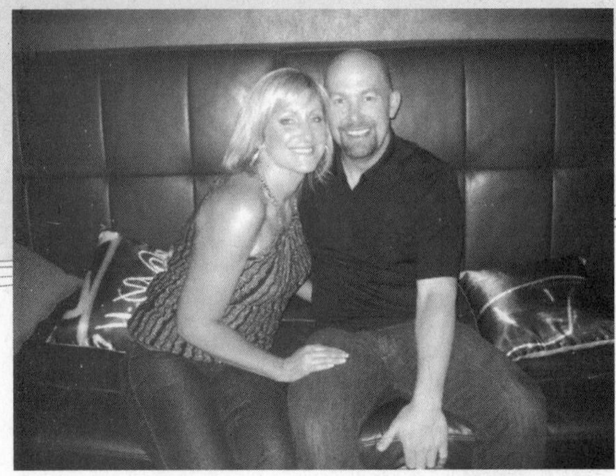

Phil and Amy,
May 2009

Amy on vacation,
2004

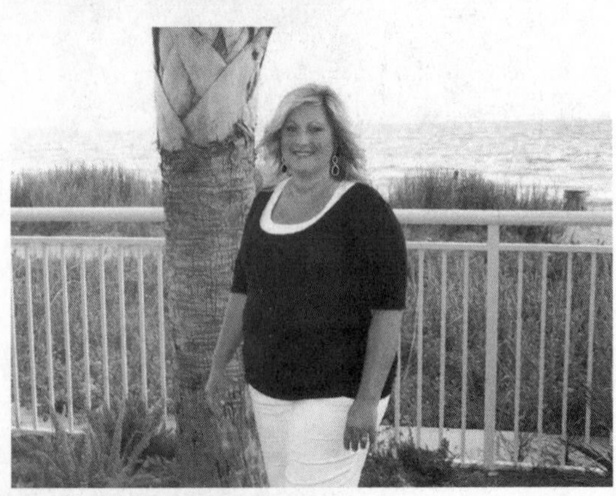

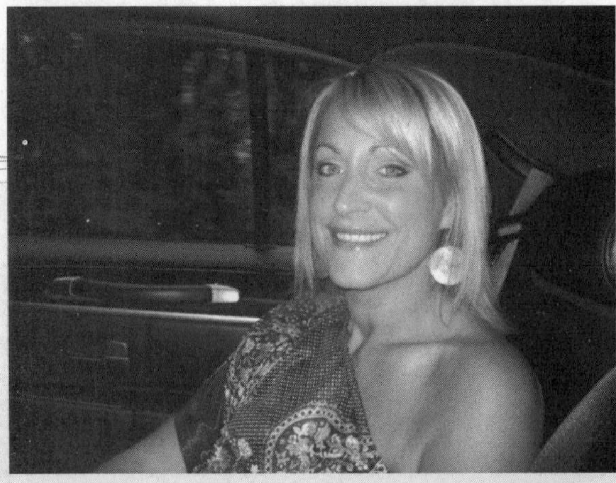

Amy today

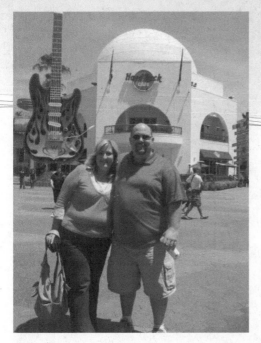

Phil and Amy in Los Angeles, May 2008

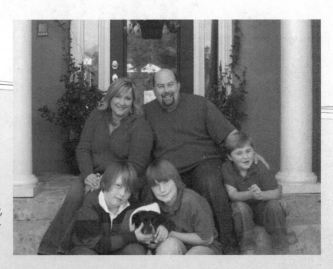

The Parham family, Christmas 2007

Our boys
(from l to r: Pearson, Rhett, and Austin)

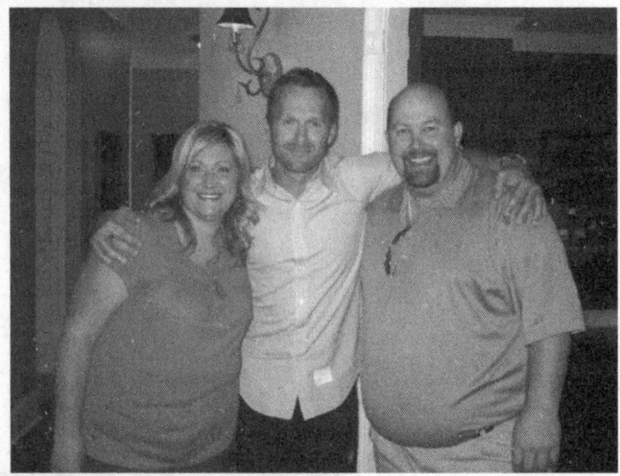

Phil and Amy with Bob Harper, May 2008. Time for change!

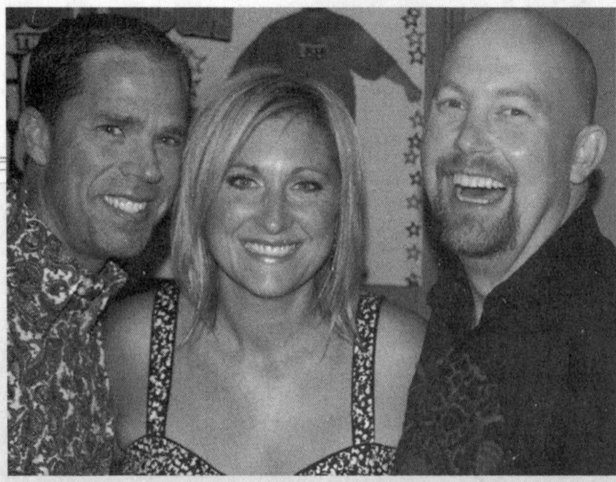

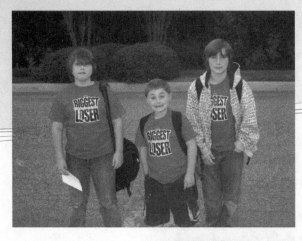

Phil and Amy with their trainer, D.J., September 2008

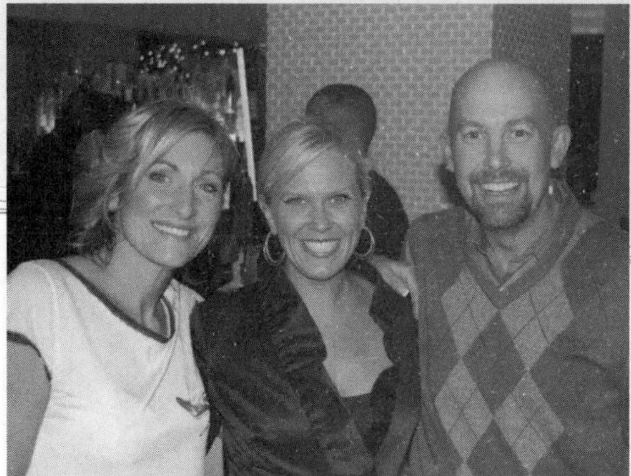

Phil and Amy with Julie Hadden, December 2008, after the show's finale

The new Phil!

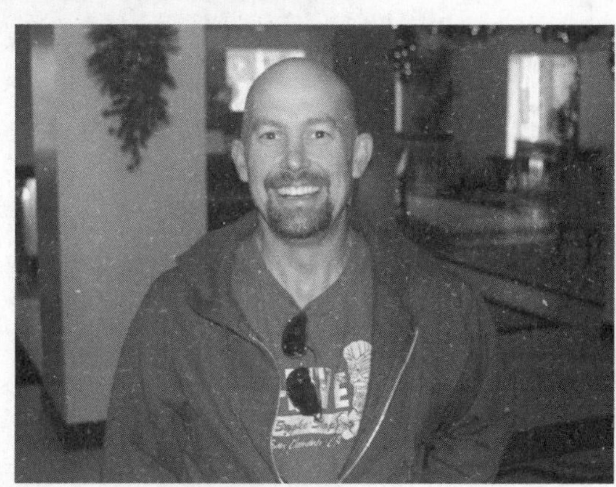

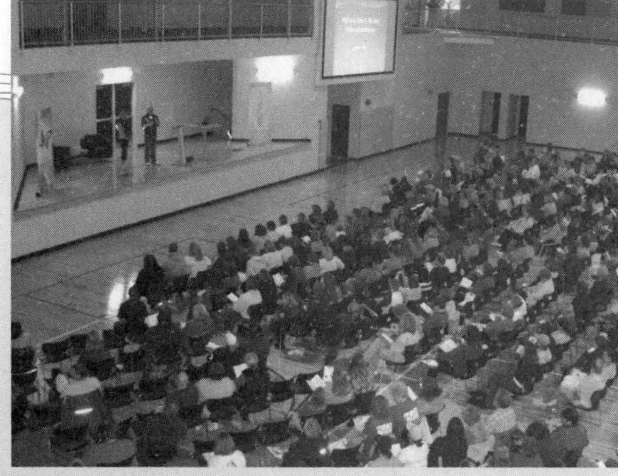

Speaking at our first "Challenge" event, January 2009

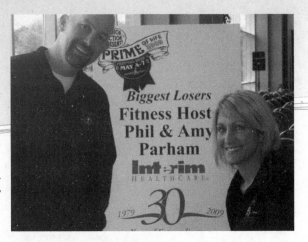

Phil and Amy hosting a "Challenge" event for seniors

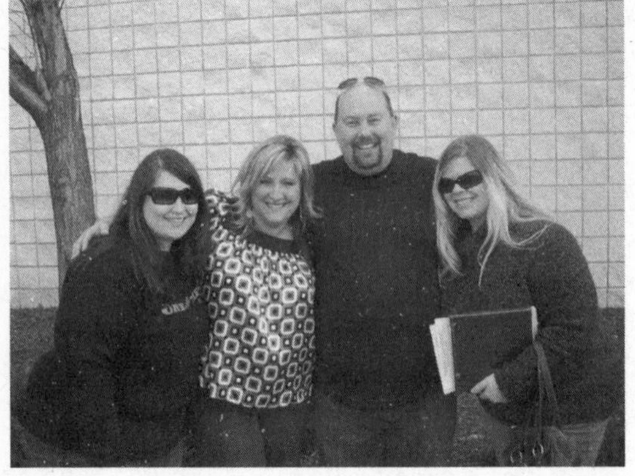

From l. to r.:
Lolo, Amy, Phil, and Rae at the casting call

Part 2

Your Daily Fitness Challenge

For the next ninety days, we are going to walk with you each day as you progress on this fitness journey. You'll learn, be inspired, and get challenged as you make your way toward better health.

Let's take a quick refresher course. You now know how to eat to live. Stick with foods that are whole and natural—fruits, vegetables, nuts, and lean meats. Stay away from processed or packaged products and foods that contain a lot of sugar and salt. Don't forget to balance all your meals with protein, carbohydrates, and healthy fats. Eat your fiber so your body can be regularly cleansed of toxins and impurities and leave you feeling energized and good all day long. Keep the water bottle handy and guzzle water all day long.

We don't want you to go crazy counting calories, but try not to exceed the number of calories you need to help you lose weight slowly, steadily, and healthily. If you don't know how many calories are in what foods, check out the *CalorieKing Calorie, Fat, and Carbohydrate Counter* to learn more. If you are feeling tired, cranky, moody, depressed, or upset, don't use food to try to make you feel better. Eat only to fuel your body and give it proper running power. Don't eat to fulfill an emotional need; eat to live.

You also know you need to get moving and activate your body. The important thing is to be physically active daily—whether that means raking leaves, playing with your kids in the backyard, going for a walk around the block, or hitting the gym. Sometimes all you have to do is just get off the couch. Substitute any kind of movement for a sedentary lifestyle.

Follow our three-tier fitness plan in appendix E, which will provide you with some great fat-blasting cardio and strength-training exercises. Every thirty days, your plan will change to a little more intense one. After all, as times goes by, you will be losing weight, feeling better, and getting stronger. If you want to follow a different exercise routine, go to your local library or bookstore and check out the following books to help you on your way:

- *The Biggest Loser Fitness Program: Fast, Safe, and Effective Workouts to Target and Tone Your Trouble Spots—Adapted from NBC's Hit Show!* by *The Biggest Loser* experts and cast, with Maggie Greenwood-Robinson
- *Shape Magazine's Ultimate Body Book: 4 Weeks to Your Best Abs, Butt, Thighs, and More* by Linda Shelton with Angela Hynes
- *Fitness for Dummies* by Suzanne Schlosberg and Liz Neporent

Throughout this challenge, we will be right by your side as you move into a new, healthier you. Each day will be a new adventure where you will learn more and feel better about yourself. Every day for the next ninety days, we will present you with

- some inspiring thoughts to help you get through the day
- health tips, because taking care of ourselves is a constant learning process
- space to write down your food and calorie intake (remember how important food journaling is) as well as your exercise
- journaling space for you to write down some of your thoughts (you might want to get a separate notebook if you need more space)

These daily fitness challenges are divided into eleven segments over the ninety days. The final devotion in each segment is a success story, an email we've received from someone who has participated in the "Challenge." We are confident these stories will encourage you as you "write" your own. If you want to be further inspired and encouraged, go to philandamyfitness.com and create a profile where you can share your journey with others who are on the same path. You might even find a support group in your area.

One last thing. We are so proud you've decided to start this journey with us. We know you can accomplish all your goals. Go to appendix A and look at where you are. Remind yourself of your goals and where you want to be ninety days from now.

We know you can do this. We know you can meet your goals. We know you can change your life for the better and forever. You are on the road to better health, and before you know it, you will start seeing some changes in your health, body, and mind that will just amaze you. Get ready to see some lasting and mind-blowing results!

Now let's get started.

Dream About What You Want Your Life to Be

The "90-Day Fitness Challenge" is about dreaming, believing, and achieving. We begin by helping you reflect on your dreams and setting goals for the next ninety days. You will recognize the importance of making your health a priority. By the end of the week, you will have fresh inspiration to create a better future knowing that all is possible.

DAY 1—DREAM A LITTLE DREAM

"For I know the plans I have for you," declares the LORD,
"plans to prosper you and not to harm you,
plans to give you hope and a future."
JEREMIAH 29:11 NIV

A Word from Amy

When you were a little kid, did you dream of having an average, mediocre, or boring life? I suspect not. When I was a little girl I wanted to be just like Loretta Lynn. I would stand in the living room and sing "Coal Miner's Daughter" at the top of my lungs, pretending to be her. My dad was a radio announcer, and when I turned six, he gave me the best surprise. He took me to a country music show where I had the opportunity to go backstage and meet my idol. Loretta even let me sit on her lap while she waited to go on stage. I will never forget that day. I remember every detail of it, even what she was wearing.

Unfortunately, I was no Loretta Lynn. I couldn't sing at all. So I let go of that dream and moved on to other things. But I never stopped dreaming.

Early in our lives most of us dream big dreams. We want to do things that seem impossible. We want to live a life that contributes to mankind in an important way.

I am convinced that we allow setbacks in life to cause us to stop dreaming. When we experience heartbreak or difficulty, our inclination is to protect ourselves by not trying to reach a goal or commit to something that might bring us pain again. My challenge to you today is to not give up; keep your dream alive. If you got knocked down, it's time to get back up. If you failed many times with getting fit, it's time to try one more time.

I know it can be easy to get stuck in a routine, especially if you've lost your desire to dream. And let's be honest. Sometimes life can be mundane and boring, the same old stuff day in and day out. Don't let life get you down; it can become exciting once again. Remember where Phil and I were and where we are today. Our lives have completely changed, and yours can too.

Mini-Challenge of the Day

Think about some dreams you may have had that have disappeared or are stored away somewhere in your heart. What do you still dream you can become or do with your life? This can be about your weight-loss goals or something unrelated to your health, such as starting a new business, learning a new hobby, or getting a master's degree. Whatever your desires, write them down on a piece of paper and put it where you can see it and be reminded each day.

Tip of the Day

Studies have shown that people who write down their dreams or goals have an 80 percent greater chance of achieving them. Grab a bunch of Post-it notes and write something on them that relates to your dream. You can write down whatever you want as long as it is goal-oriented and centers on your desires. Then put them all over your home, your car, or at work. Seeing them written down will encourage you to keep on going.

Meal	Record Your Food & Water Intake for the Day	Calories
1		
2		
3		
4		
5		
	Total Calories	

Fitness Plan

Cardio activity: ____________________ Time: ________ Miles: ______

Intensity level (circle one): L M H

Strength training (circle): Lower body Upper body Core

My Thoughts

____

____

____

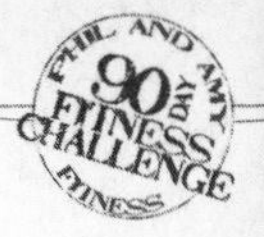

DAY 2—TIME IS ON YOUR SIDE

"There is no time like the present."

A Note from Phil

Often, we don't rise to meet challenges because of the time it will take to finish the task. Many things we want to do take a lot of work and usually more time than we anticipate. This can be very frustrating. Here's a little secret: time moves on with or without you.

A coworker once told me he wished he was brave enough to leave his current job and attend medical school. Being a doctor was this man's lifelong goal, but it would take a lot of time to get there—eight years of schooling and residency. This was much too long for him, so he chose to keep his job and forget about his dream. Thirteen years have passed since that conversation. I've often thought about how his life would have been different had he pursued his goal. This man would be in his fifth year of practice as a physician, but instead he continues working at that same job. Time will pass whether you accomplish your goals or not.

When we were on the ranch, all of us on the show dropped a tremendous amount of weight in what seemed like a short time. Viewers at home were excited because of what they thought were fast results. That wasn't the case, of course. It took us a lot of time and hard work to lose weight, certainly more time than the thirty minutes shown on TV once a week. Some days we were exercising up to eight hours a day!

Now is the time to remind yourself that you did not put on all your weight in three months, so you can't expect it all to come off in three months. If you consistently stick to the program, in time you will reach your dream of being fit and thin. It will just take time, maybe even a little longer than you expect. The most important thing to keep in mind is that in the next ninety days, you will make incredible progress and be well on your way to reaching your goals. Those ninety days will pass whether you choose to reach your goals. Be inspired to be fit and healthy in three months.

Mini-Challenge of the Day

Promise yourself to live one day at a time. (On some days it'll be one hour at a time.) If you do this, eventually you will reach your goals.

Tip of the Day

Find a Bible verse or positive affirmation that is inspiring and meaningful to your life. Memorize it and say it out loud every morning after you brush your teeth. Here is an example: "It's more stressful to continue being fat than to stop overeating." Keep positive.

Meal	Record Your Food & Water Intake for the Day	Calories
1		
2		
3		
4		
5		
	Total Calories	

Fitness Plan

Cardio activity: ____________________ Time: ________ Miles: ______

Intensity level (circle one): L M H

Strength training (circle): Lower body Upper body Core

My Thoughts

____

____

____

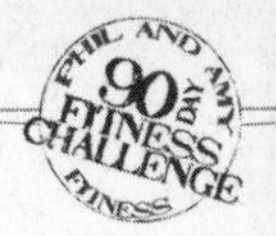

DAY 3—LOSE THE GUILT

"Here's the one important thing to remember with oxygen masks. Put your mask on first before doing anything for anyone else."
TheTravelInsider.info, "How to Survive a Plane Crash"

A Word from Amy

When you fly on an airplane, the flight attendant always tells you that in the case of an emergency, you must put on your oxygen mask first before you help the person next to you, even if it's your own child. It seems backward as most of us are used to putting others before ourselves. But how are you going to help the person next to you if you are unable to breathe yourself?

Women are especially notorious for doing everything for everyone else and putting themselves on the back burner. What I have learned from talking to people all over the country is that there is a universal feeling of guilt when we care for our needs. Many of us feel guilty all the time. I truly believe guilt is a wasted emotion. Feeling guilty doesn't change a single thing.

One thing that I hope you lose in this challenge, besides weight, is the guilt associated with taking time for yourself. You must take time for you. You must take the time to exercise, to cook your meals, to recharge by getting adequate sleep. You must take the time to love yourself. You must have your own identity and remember who you are. You are more than a spouse or a parent or a friend or a sibling. You must make yourself healthy and happy first before you can really help others.

As children we dream of what we're going to do or be when we grow up. As we get older we have so much to do that sometimes our dreams get lost in the shuffle. Don't let this happen to you. Realize that taking time for you is a good thing. It helps you to have the energy and stability of mind to take care of the ones you love. Exercise produces chemicals in the brain that fight depression and help to ease anxiety. Rest helps your body to recover so you can deal with the stresses of life. God rested on the seventh day for a reason. He was setting an example for us to follow because He made our bodies and He knows what is best for them.

Make time for you a priority today.

Mini-Challenge of the Day

Block out at least three to four times a week for exercise. Put this in your calendar and organize your day around this time. If you have children, most fitness centers provide childcare. If not, exercise when your kids are in school or find a neighbor or friend who understands how much this health journey means to you and ask if she can watch them for a while. You have to find the time to make working out a priority. It just might save your life.

Tip of the Day

When shopping, park in the parking space farthest from the entrance instead of driving around to find the closest spot. Make this a habit every time you go shopping. You will burn calories and get some well-needed fresh air.

Meal	Record Your Food & Water Intake for the Day	Calories
1		
2		
3		
4		
5		
	Total Calories	

Fitness Plan

Cardio activity: ____________________ Time: _______ Miles: _____

Intensity level (circle one): L M H

Strength training (circle): Lower body Upper body Core

My Thoughts

____

____

____

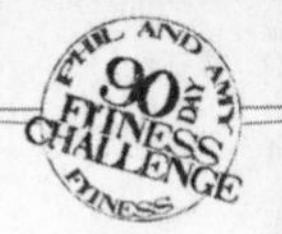

DAY 4—DREAMS AND VISIONS

"The secret to productive goal setting is in establishing clearly defined goals, writing them down and then focusing on them several times a day with words, pictures and emotions as if we've already achieved them."

Denis Waitley

A Note from Phil

The Bible says that in the last days God will pour His Spirit out on all flesh and that young men will see visions and old men will dream dreams (Acts 2:17). Why do you suppose the young men are the ones seeing the visions? Why not the middle-aged or seniors? I believe it is because you have to have a vision (early) before you can dream the dream (later). I like to think of a vision as a plan. It is how you see yourself getting to where you want to go.

For example, you may want to write a book one day, but to make that dream come true you have to map out a plan of action. You have to have an idea. You have to write a book proposal. You may want to get a literary agent. And, of course, you have to actually write a book. Then when all the steps are finished, you have a dream that is realized.

We have talked about dreaming about what you want your life to be, but in order for your dreams to happen you have to have a specific vision. You have to create a plan. You have to list objectives. And you have to commit to meeting your goals.

Take the time and ask God what His purpose is for your life. You probably already have a hint because His plan always fulfills your very deepest desires, desires that He has already placed in your heart. Doing what He has called you to do means you are going to be fulfilled. As you pray, ask Him for the steps to fulfill that dream. And spend time doing your own research. See what steps you need to climb to get where you want to go. These steps will be your vision. Walk out that vision and live your dreams.

Mini-Challenge of the Day

If you are reading this book, we both already know that one of your dreams is to be fitter and healthier in ninety days. In the journal space, write down five mini-goals of how you will get there. For example, if you want to lose twenty pounds, how will you do that? What mini-goals will you need to accomplish every day in order to meet the ninety-day goal? Begin with "I will..."

____

____

____

Tip of the Day

Sometimes we can sabotage our own success. It's hard to do something challenging on our own. We can become discouraged. The journey might be lonely. We may think that no one understands what we are going through. In these moments you need support. Many local churches and communities offer faith-based support groups for weight loss. Check your local paper and see if there is one in your area you can join.

Meal	Record Your Food & Water Intake for the Day	Calories
1		
2		
3		
4		
5		
	Total Calories	

Fitness Plan

Cardio activity: ______________ Time: ________ Miles: ______

Intensity level (circle one): L M H

Strength training (circle): Lower body Upper body Core

My Thoughts

____

____

____

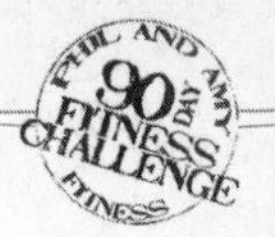

DAY 5—FAITH MATTERS

"Now faith is the substance of things hoped for, the evidence of things not seen."
HEBREWS 11:1 NKJV

A Word from Amy

What do you think about when you read the above verse? Do you get it? Does it make sense? Or does it sound like a riddle or a mystery? I was confused about this verse for a long time. Since faith is intangible, how can it be the "substance of things hoped for"? And since you can't see faith, how can it be "evidence"?

One pastor helped me to understand this verse by likening the faith in your heart to a blueprint for what you want. Let's say you want to own your dream home. The blueprint is not the house, but it is the evidence that you plan to build a house. It is the guide that shows you in great detail what the finished product is going to look like.

What is faith? Faith believes without a shadow of doubt that the dream in your heart will happen. You may have been too afraid to believe for big things for your life. You may have tried and failed before. You may have been disappointed by other people letting you down. I encourage you today to never give up the faith. The Bible tells us that "without faith it is impossible to please Him, for he who comes to God must believe that He is, and that He is a rewarder of those who diligently seek Him" (Hebrews 11:6 NKJV). So go diligently toward your dreams and have faith.

You might not know what your body will look like after you lose thirty or fifty pounds. So many of us have been overweight for so long, we cannot even grasp what it's like to live like a thin person. Let faith fuel you to picture yourself as a thin person. Let faith fuel you to picture yourself finally fitting into your old clothes. Let faith fuel you to picture yourself running around with your kids on the playground. Maybe you have only a little bit of faith right now and can't fully fathom reaching your dream weight. Just focus on a smaller goal, such as losing ten or twenty pounds. The closer you get to your goal, the more your faith will stretch. Don't give up!

Mini-Challenge of the Day

Faith works by love so if you have unforgiveness in your heart toward anyone today, release that burden so God can work in your life. Write a letter to the person who has hurt you (you don't have to mail it if you don't want to). If you feel the need, you can pick up the phone and call them, or just release this burden silently from your heart. The less emotional baggage you have, the easier it will be to focus on losing the physical weight.

Tip of the Day

Do you need some inspiration or motivation while you work out? Try an audio book or download a faith message onto your iPod. It will give you the strength to keep on striving toward your dream.

Meal	Record Your Food & Water Intake for the Day	Calories
1		
2		
3		
4		
5		
	Total Calories	

Fitness Plan

Cardio activity: ____________________ Time: ________ Miles: _____

Intensity level (circle one): L M H

Strength training (circle): Lower body Upper body Core

My Thoughts

____

____

____

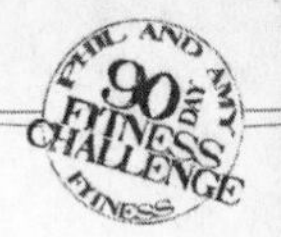

DAY 6—NEW THRILLS

"I can do all things through Christ who strengthens me."
PHILIPPIANS 4:13 NKJV

A Note from Phil

When I got back from *The Biggest Loser* campus, I went on a vacation with my family to Pigeon Forge, Tennessee. One of the things we wanted to do was visit the Dollywood Theme Park. Before my weight loss, I hated theme parks. I would find any reason why I couldn't go. All I could think about was the walking, the sweating, the lines, the people, and that I didn't fit on any of the cool rides.

I remember going to a local amusement park and wanting to ride the go-carts with my sons. I found myself making excuses about why we should play miniature golf instead. Secretly I was scared I wouldn't fit in the cart or that I would get stuck in the seat and embarrass my kids. My life once again was dictated to me by my weight. I avoided amusement parks at all costs.

Now here I was at Dollywood with my family as a thinner man. This time was different. I was excited about going to the theme park because we were going to walk and do fun things. It was a great feeling to know I was burning calories and having fun at the same time (that's how much my mentality had changed). I could not wait to get on the roller coaster and even considered bungee jumping.

Only three months after my transformation, I was looking at life from a completely new perspective. I was starting to live again. Not only did I have a great time at Dollywood that day with my family, with my new mindset I started to think of other things I could do. I started talking about going water skiing. I started dreaming of big and small things I could do that would continue to make my life fun.

You too can experience the joys of fulfilling the dreams of your life, even the things you were never able to do before or haven't done in a while. Life will become fun again for you. Always keep the dreams alive in your heart. You *will* get there!

Mini-Challenge of the Day

Write down one activity you have avoided doing because of your weight. Describe why you have avoided it and how it made you feel. Now imagine how it would feel to do that activity with the new you, thinner and full of energy.

Write down as many details as you can below. Ninety days from now, this will be the new you!

____

____

____

Tip of the Day

Find a picture of a healthy and thin person that is inspiring to you. It could be an athlete from a magazine, or even a photo of you when you were thinner. Be realistic about this. Don't choose a picture from when you were thin at thirteen or of an anorexic model in a magazine. The picture should make you feel good and excited about what you can achieve in the next ninety days. Tape this photo to your fridge so you can see it every day.

Meal	Record Your Food & Water Intake for the Day	Calories
1		
2		
3		
4		
5		
	Total Calories	

Fitness Plan

Cardio activity: ______________ Time: ________ Miles: ______

Intensity level (circle one): L M H

Strength training (circle): Lower body Upper body Core

My Thoughts

____

____

____

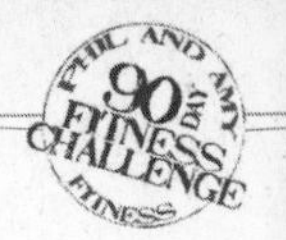

DAY 7—YOU CAN DO IT!

"If you think you can do it
or you think you can't do it, you are right."
HENRY FORD

Esther is a beautiful young mom who let life and the responsibilities of taking care of others overwhelm her. She was so busy tending to everyone else that her health fell by the wayside. When we met her for the first time at one of our "Challenge" events, Esther seemed quiet and shy. We had no idea how emotional that day was for her. When you read her story below, you will find out what changed in her life.

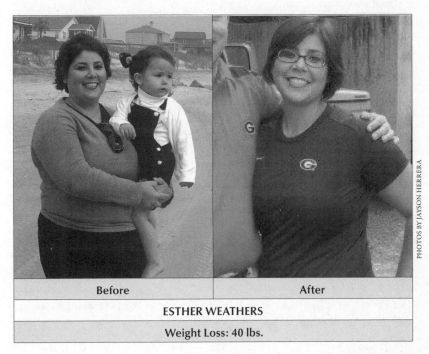

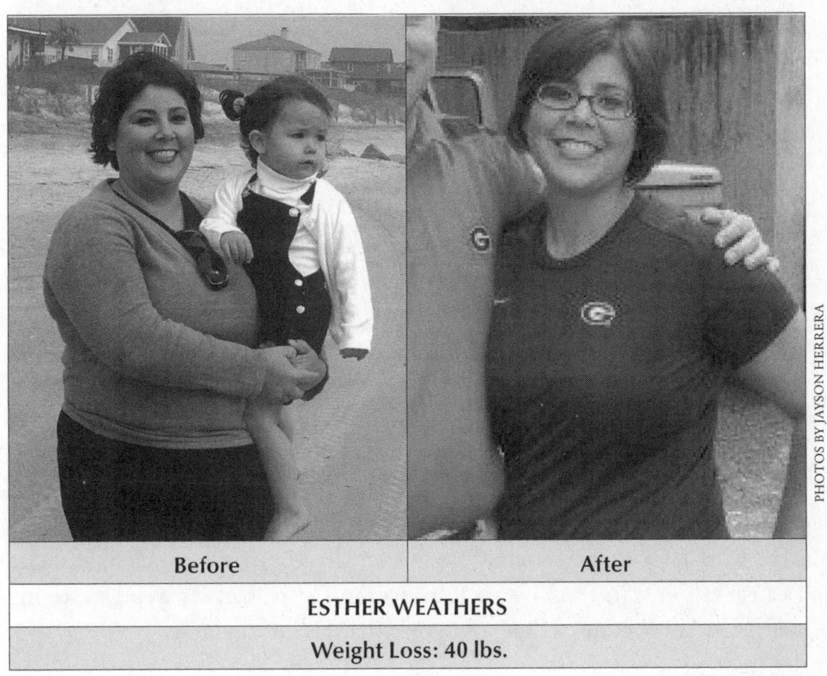

Before	After
ESTHER WEATHERS	
Weight Loss: 40 lbs.	

PHOTOS BY JAYSON HERRERA

"In the past nine years, I've slowly gained eighty-five pounds. I struggled with my weight but never dealt with it because I was too busy with my life and my family. A year ago, I went to a children's gym called Pump-It-Up with my beautiful daughter, Isabel. I was so out of shape, it was a struggle for me to do all the activities with her. I was so embarrassed by how red and sweaty I got and by how much trouble I had breathing. I decided I needed to get in shape.

"I hired a personal trainer, and over the next few months, I did weight training consistently. I became stronger, but I didn't lose any weight. My trainer told me there are three keys to weight loss: eating right, cardio, and weight training. I was missing two of the three keys. I almost never did any cardio and my food habits were horrible. Even though I knew this, I still didn't make any permanent changes.

"At the end of December 2008, my husband and I took our daughter to the beach. I thought it would be fun to take some pictures. Little did I know this would be the catalyst for losing weight. Days later, when I saw myself in the pictures, I cried and literally felt sick to my stomach. I thought I looked like Jabba the Hutt in the *Star Wars* movies. I hit rock bottom. How had I not noticed how large I was?

"I found out about the '90-Day Fitness Challenge' from a coworker a few weeks afterward. She helped give me the courage to go to the event once I learned there wouldn't be a public weigh-in. I refused to share my weight with anyone except my doctor. After the 'Challenge,' I measured and weighed myself at home. More tears. The reality of how much I weighed and my waist measurement was so embarrassing. I couldn't believe just nine years ago I had a 28-inch waist. I felt hideous about my weight gain.

"I realized I was an emotional eater. I had to learn to deal with my emotions without depending on food to make me feel better. I had to change my negative thinking and not believing I could lose weight to thinking positively. I started working out five to six times a week using weights and doing cardio. I started eating four to five meals a day. My dear husband has been wonderful by cooking healthier and being supportive of my health goals.

"I feel so much better, stronger, and healthier than I have in years. I even took up running and joined a running club. I recently completed the USMC Mud Run in Columbia, South Carolina, and have started running in 5K races. I can't wait to start training for 10K races in December. It's weird to see my 'before' picture because I don't recognize that person anymore."

Mini-Challenge of the Day

For today, play! Find a child (yours or someone else's) and play with them for thirty minutes. Run with them, jump with them, take them to the park and chase them around. If you can't find a child, borrow a pet and do the same thing.

Tip of the Day

Did you know that the most inexpensive protein sources in the supermarket are eggs, tuna, and chicken? Remember this next time you're shopping on a budget.

Meal	Record Your Food & Water Intake for the Day	Calories
1		
2		
3		
4		
5		
	Total Calories	

Fitness Plan

Cardio activity: ____________________ Time: ________ Miles: ______

Intensity level (circle one): L M H

Strength training (circle): Lower body Upper body Core

My Thoughts

____

____

____

Recognize Where You Are Today

Over the next several days, we will help you face reality to better prepare you for your future. It's time to get weighed, get a physical, and get the right running shoes. You will also recognize that your past doesn't have to become your future. These daily challenges will surround you with a positive support system and equip you to move forward with your new "can-do" attitude.

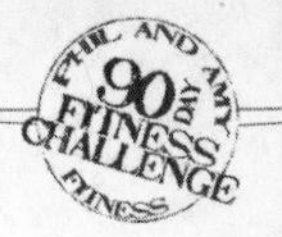

DAY 8—EXPOSING YOURSELF

"You must take personal responsibility.
You cannot change the circumstances, the seasons,
or the wind, but you can change yourself.
That is something you have charge of."

Jim Rohn

A Word from Amy

One of the first things we had to do when we were chosen for *The Biggest Loser* was the infamous photo shoot in sports bra and shorts (for guys it was just shorts). It was an intimidating moment having to walk in front of a photographer and pose with all your fat hanging out everywhere. I was quite embarrassed, but knew it had to be done. As the shoot continued, I realized that more than my body would be exposed to the world. My heart would be exposed as well. I had to be open to the entire process of losing weight so that I could make lasting changes in my life.

When you first started this challenge, we asked you to recognize where you are by weighing yourself, getting a physical checkup, and taking a "before" picture in a bathing suit. I know those were tough to do. It's never easy to face reality, especially if it doesn't look pretty. Thankfully, you don't have to publicly announce your stats and show your "before" picture to the world, but you do have to face those things for yourself.

You might be shocked at the results and want to hide from the world. You might be surprised at the numbers on the scale and realize that's why your clothes have been getting tighter. There is no need to beat yourself up about what the numbers or results look like. Remember, it's a starting point.

Taking inventory of how you have come to be overweight is very important. It's time to be honest. Maybe you struggle with eating certain foods or waking up in the middle of the night and binging. Maybe you use food to cope with stress. I encourage you to share your challenges with someone so they can help you find a solution. Hiding addictions and keeping habits a secret only gives them more power. The Bible tells us to confess our faults to one another so that we may be healed (James 5:16). I believe that showing the world my faults is what allowed me to recognize my poor health and move toward healing.

Don't be afraid to expose yourself. It will lead you to the new you.

Mini-Challenge of the Day

If you haven't done so already, make an appointment for a physical checkup. Get weighed. Then get into a bathing suit and have someone take your "before" picture. Take a good look—this is the launching pad of the "Challenge."

Tip of the Day

Always have a learning attitude. Read books and magazines about health, nutrition, and exercise. Read up on information that will help you be healthier and more fit. Check with your local library, gym, community center, and even your grocery store. Most offer free classes and workshops about health. Keep growing and learn as much as you can in your journey toward health.

Meal	Record Your Food & Water Intake for the Day	Calories
1		
2		
3		
4		
5		
	Total Calories	

Fitness Plan

Cardio activity: ______________________ Time: ________ Miles: ______

Intensity level (circle one): L M H

Strength training (circle): Lower body Upper body Core

My Thoughts

____

____

____

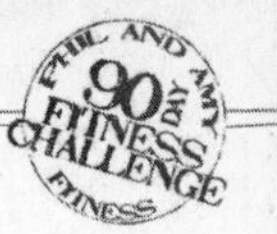

DAY 9—SUPPORT: WE ALL NEED IT

"Two are better than one
because they have a good return for their labor."
ECCLESIASTES 4:9 NASB

A Note from Phil

Many of us embark on major change thinking we should be brave and go at the challenge alone. We think all we have to do is to eat less and exercise. How hard can that be? Some of us think we will wake up one day and, like the Nike slogan, "Just do it." Sorry folks, but losing weight doesn't work that way—not if you have spent years unfit and overweight.

I was examining my life one day and realized that I had a lot of people around me who were involved in my weight-loss process. I had a doctor, a dietician, a psychologist, my wife, and my friends to support and encourage me. I was also fortunate to have an amazing trainer and coach. He would pick me up on Saturdays, and we would go hiking or run bleachers at the local high school. He held me accountable each and every day. I truly believe I would not be where I am today without his invaluable encouragement.

Now that I'm back at home, I may not have as much professional support as I had while on the show, but it doesn't matter. Amy and I still have each other and have surrounded ourselves with great local support as we continue the path to good health. If I had to do it alone, I don't think I would keep the weight off.

Everyone needs a coach. A coach is there to challenge you and push you. A great coach will help you realize your potential. I have friends who are very successful, and every time they take on a new project, they hire a coach. This is the strategy of many wealthy and successful people. Even LeBron James and Tiger Woods have coaches. They know someone else can see their weaknesses and make them better at their game. A coach can be a professional, a mentor, or even a sibling or friend who is your cheerleader during your weight-loss journey.

We need to be honest enough with ourselves to admit that we need help. We all need to be pushed to go to higher levels. Accountability can lead us to new heights. Challenge yourself today to ask for help where you need it.

Mini-Challenge of the Day

If you haven't already, find yourself a professional coach. Think of it as an investment in yourself. This could be a life coach, a dietician, or a personal trainer. It doesn't matter who it is as long as they are trained in coaching one aspect of the weight-loss journey. Even today I work with a personal trainer one day a week to keep me on track. I've decided I'm worth the investment.

Tip of the Day

Use natural sweeteners whenever possible. We stick with Stevia and Xylitol. These are the ones we feel the best about because they have a natural base. From our experience, natural is always better than artificial.

Meal	Record Your Food & Water Intake for the Day	Calories
1		
2		
3		
4		
5		
	Total Calories	

Fitness Plan

Cardio activity: ____________________ Time: ________ Miles: _____

Intensity level (circle one): L M H

Strength training (circle): Lower body Upper body Core

My Thoughts

____

____

____

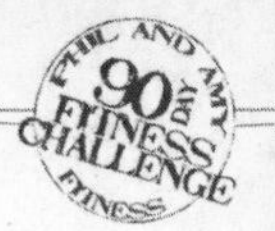

DAY 10—REGAINING CONTROL

"Don't be afraid to give your best
to what seemingly are small jobs.
Every time you conquer one
it makes you that much stronger.
If you do the little jobs well,
the big ones will tend to take care of themselves."
Dale Carnegie

A Note from Phil

It's amazing how getting one aspect of your life under control makes you think of other areas that are out of control. As I got a handle on my weight, I looked around and saw other things in my life that needed work. I had to recognize where I was and how I was doing in areas such as family, career, and finances, and ask myself if I was happy with the way things were going. In many cases the answer was no.

I realized some of the same strategies I applied to accomplish my weight-loss goals would help me achieve goals in other life areas. For example, when I started losing weight I decided to practice finishing what I started. If I told myself that I would spend one hour on the treadmill, then I was going to stay on for an hour, no matter what. I set goals, had ups and downs, and pushed myself to new levels.

I realized that procrastination had stopped me from losing weight sooner in my life. Now it was affecting the rest of me. I did not like the way I would procrastinate about ideas I had for my life, about things I needed to change in my business, and about decisions that I didn't want to make. I figured out that if I set mini-goals and achieved them (just as I did on the ranch), then I could stop procrastinating and start accomplishing.

This challenge is about a whole lot more than weight. There is a whole new world waiting for you. A new world in your career, your family, your friends, even in your community. Getting good at the little things will help you tackle the bigger things. Before you know it, you have a whole new life.

Mini-Challenge of the Day

What are some areas in your life that need extra attention? Work? Finances? Relationships? Write down a list of things you would like to improve. Don't try to fix everything in ninety days. As long as you have written them down, you are aware of them. You can tackle them one at a time when you are ready.

____

____

____

____

Tip of the Day

Are you sleeping enough? Most experts say that getting seven to eight hours a night is vital to your health and well-being. I know the "90-Day Fitness Challenge" is tough, so you need this recovery time more than ever. Sleep is where your body and your mind recharge. Make sure you are getting plenty of *z*'s.

Meal	Record Your Food & Water Intake for the Day	Calories
1		
2		
3		
4		
5		
	Total Calories	

Fitness Plan

Cardio activity: ____________________ Time: ________ Miles: ______

Intensity level (circle one): L M H

Strength training (circle): Lower body Upper body Core

My Thoughts

____

____

____

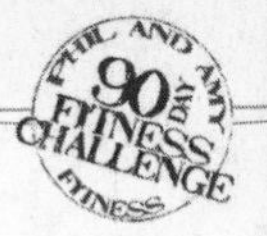

DAY 11—**DON'T GET "DEFEETED"**

"Forewarned, forearmed; to be prepared is half the victory."
Miguel de Cervantes Saavedra, Spanish writer

A Word from Amy

I remember when Phil and I finally decided it was time to get some new running shoes. While we were on the show, our footwear was provided for us, and we never had to think about what we needed to wear and why. We loved that. Before we became "athletes," we would go to any shoe store and ask for a shoe that we liked or was on sale. If it came in our size, great. That was the only criteria we used. We never had our feet evaluated by a professional athletic shoe specialist. We didn't even know there was such a thing.

When we got to the store, the salesperson asked me to take off my shoes and socks and step on a foot measurer. He measured my foot not only while I was standing but also while I had my foot resting at an angle without weight on it. This gentleman performed more tests to determine the type of arch I had, the size of my feet, and the support I needed. Finally, he showed me the shoes in the store that would work for my specific foot needs. I never knew each person's feet were so unique.

Picking the right running shoes is a science. I learned that if I didn't wear the right shoe, I would be prone to discomfort and injury. Shin splints, knee problems, hip strains, and stress fractures—all these ailments can be related to wearing the wrong shoe. If we are hurt, then we are less likely to continue with our exercise routine. If it's bad enough, we might not be able to work out at all. Also, shoes that don't fit properly will cause blisters, which I know from experience are no fun.

When I went to the store, I learned the importance of choosing the right footwear for running. And boy did I notice a difference. My runs with my new shoes were so much better and more comfortable.

Mini-Challenge of the Day

Part of recognizing where you are today is looking at what you have and figuring out what you need. If you don't have the right shoes, then you're in trouble. Get out to a local athletic store and invest in a good pair of cross-training, aerobic, walking, or running shoes. Get your shoes professionally selected for you.

Tip of the Day

Invest in a good set of plastic storage containers or Tupperware. You can cook on the weekends and be prepared for the week or store extras from dinner for lunch the next day. It makes planning meals a lot easier.

Meal	Record Your Food & Water Intake for the Day	Calories
1		
2		
3		
4		
5		
	Total Calories	

Fitness Plan

Cardio activity: ______________________ Time: ________ Miles: ______

Intensity level (circle one): L M H

Strength training (circle): Lower body Upper body Core

My Thoughts

____

____

____

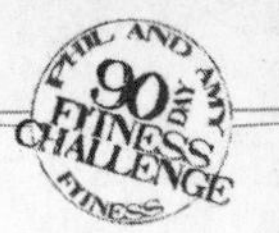

DAY 12—CAN-DO WORDS

"If there is a will, there is a way."

Old English Proverb

A Note from Phil

Our public weight-loss journey has opened up opportunities to speak to people all around the country. We've given countless lectures and talks and have spent hours listening and talking with participants in the "Challenge." When I was in college, one of my Bible instructors told me that you can know a person's character by what comes out of his mouth. If you really listen to someone, you can tell what is in his heart and what he believes.

After listening to thousands of people struggling on their weight-loss journey, I noticed a pattern. Their sentences would start with "I can't" or "I don't." "I can't give up my sodas." "I can't work out because I don't have time." "I don't have the money to eat healthy." They spend half of our conversation telling me why they can't lose weight. They are defeated before they even begin!

A friend of mine told me a story about his third-grade teacher. She told her class to write the words "I can't" on a piece of paper, then she took them outside where they saw a hole in the ground next to a shovel. She told them the words "I can't" should never be part of their vocabulary because it would always limit them. You can guess what the hole was for. One by one, they put their paper in the hole and then watched as their teacher covered them with dirt. They made a vow that day never to say the words "I can't" again. My friend never forgot that day; it changed his life.

You need to pay attention to the words that come out of your mouth. You might be used to speaking negatively, so it will probably take some effort to begin to change that. The first step is just to notice when you say "I can't" or "I don't." When you realize what you are saying, stop talking until you can find a way to start your sentence with "I can." Start thinking about the things you can do instead of the things you can't do. Remember, you can do all things through Christ who gives you strength (Philippians 4:19).

Mini-Challenge of the Day

Write down two reasons why you "can't" do something on this weight-loss challenge. For example, "I can't eat vegetables." Now change it to an "I can" sentence and give yourself a plan on how you can accomplish what you thought you could not do before. Then do it! Remember, if there is a will, there is a way.

Tip of the Day

A delicious fat-free and natural dessert is frozen grapes. You will be amazed at how satisfying these tasty treats can be after dinner. We always keep plenty stocked in our freezer.

Meal	Record Your Food & Water Intake for the Day	Calories
1		
2		
3		
4		
5		
	Total Calories	

Fitness Plan

Cardio activity: ____________________ Time: ________ Miles: ______

Intensity level (circle one): L M H

Strength training (circle): Lower body Upper body Core

My Thoughts

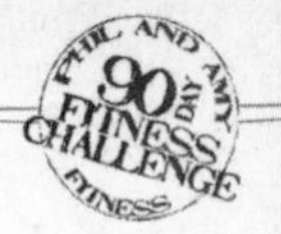

DAY 13—DON'T LOOK BACK

"You can clutch the past so tightly to your chest that it leaves your arms too full to embrace the present."
Jan Glidewell

A Word from Amy

I am a child of the '80s. My favorite song the summer after I graduated from high school was "Boys of Summer" by Don Henley. That summer, my friends and I rode a convertible down to Myrtle Beach for our graduation trip. We all wore our Ray-Ban "Wayfarer" sunglasses and thought we looked so cool. We felt as though we would never get old or have a care in the world. Guess what? We did get older and life became a lot more complicated.

A line in that song reminds us not to look back, "those days are gone forever." How many times do we look back at our life and regret decisions we made? How many times do we beat ourselves up because we think we could have done this better or not done that at all? The time we spend thinking about what might have been is time wasted. We can't afford to look back with regrets. It's pointless. We can never change anything that happened yesterday.

I spoke with a friend the other day who was upset because she had not lost enough weight before an important event and therefore had decided not to go. She was kicking herself saying, "If only I had started sooner." (Actually, she has lost about forty pounds and looks awesome. I wish she had gone to that event because I think she would have had a great time.)

In the past five years Phil and I have had the opportunity to have a lot of regrets. We lost a business and had borrowed money from relatives. We have had to work hard to financially catch up and survive, and so we have lost precious time with our children. We didn't take care of our bodies and lost out on years that we could have been living more abundant lives. At times I let myself go back to that dark place and throw myself a pity party. But I'm quick to tell myself to snap out of it!

Don't get depressed when you recognize where you are physically in this journey. Use that realization to do better and move on. There is no room in life for looking back. We only have today, and we need to make the most of it. Let's look forward with excitement for the things that are ahead. Let's take advantage of the things we've been given and enjoy them. Life is too short to live in the past. Live in the moment and never look back.

Mini-Challenge of the Day

Think about something that you regret doing or not doing that has influenced your present-day actions. Maybe you're still mourning a failed marriage you feel you are responsible for. Maybe you couldn't get into a particular school because you didn't study hard enough. Make a vow today before God that you will not allow those regrets to dictate your future. It's time to say goodbye to yesterday.

Tip of the Day

Always look at the calorie count on what you drink. Watch out for coffee beverages that just pile on the sugar. Stick with water as much as you can.

Meal	Record Your Food & Water Intake for the Day	Calories
1		
2		
3		
4		
5		
	Total Calories	

Fitness Plan

Cardio activity: ____________________ Time: ________ Miles: ______

Intensity level (circle one): L M H

Strength training (circle): Lower body Upper body Core

My Thoughts

____

____

____

DAY 14—IT IS POSSIBLE

"Optimism is the faith that leads to achievement. Nothing can be done without hope and confidence."
HELEN KELLER

Stacy Long has been an inspiration to us. We have seen her make such drastic changes in her life and have witnessed her dramatic results. She's proof that anyone can lose weight and feel better about themselves. Here is her story.

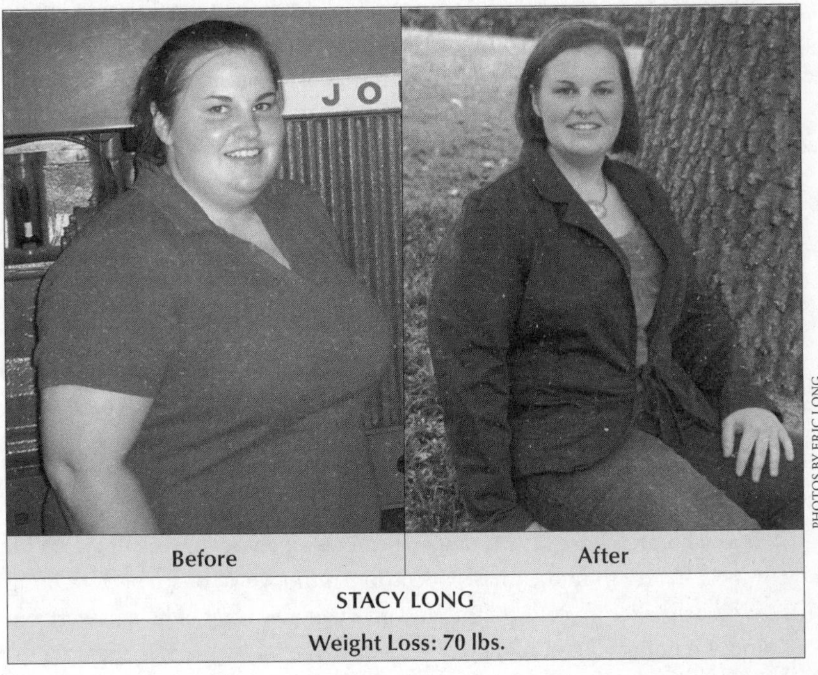

Before	After
STACY LONG	
Weight Loss: 70 lbs.	

PHOTOS BY ERIC LONG

"I started putting on weight after high school. I had gone to a boarding school and returned home to attend college. It was a big transition for me to go from living in the dorms with all of my friends to having none of them around. Sports were also a big deal for me in high school. I played volleyball, basketball, and lived for softball. After trying out for the college softball team and not making it, I was heartbroken. I turned to food for comfort and gained 60 pounds in two years.

"During my family's vacation to Orlando in January 2009, I had a major wake-up call. While at Universal Studios, I had to be moved from a regular seat on the roller coaster to a larger one. I was mortified! I was only twenty years old and could not fit in the regular seats of an amusement park ride. That was the moment I realized my weight was holding me back and something had to change. When I got home, I stepped on the scale and could not believe I weighed 260 pounds!

"My transformation started slowly. My sister Amy and I began to walk thirty minutes a day and to change our eating habits for the better. After about a month of walking, I decided to join a gym. I lost about 25 pounds and started to look for motivation to lose even more weight.

"That's when I got connected with the '90-Day Fitness Challenge.' Getting daily emails from Amy and Phil was just the motivation I needed to keep going. With the help and support of family and friends, I have lost 45 more pounds and have gone from a size 22 to a size 14.

"Thanks to Amy and Phil, I have lost a total of 70 pounds, and the athlete in me is back. I love my new lifestyle and enjoy going to the gym daily. I have run a 5K race, an 8K, and a 10K. I look forward to training for a half marathon."

Mini-Challenge of the Day

Do you have a basketball handy? If not, ask a neighbor who has kids if you can borrow their basketball. Dribble the ball for ten minutes. It's a fun activity, something new, and it will help improve your coordination. You'll have a new appreciation for basketball players.

Tip of the Day

Many libraries have DVDs that you can check out for a week or two. Visit your local library to find exercise videos for cardio, yoga, or strength training. This will help spice up your routine and give you new ideas of how to work out without spending a lot of money.

Meal	Record Your Food & Water Intake for the Day	Calories
1		
2		
3		
4		
5		
	Total Calories	

Fitness Plan

Cardio activity: ____________________ Time: ________ Miles: ______

Intensity level (circle one): L M H

Strength training (circle): Lower body Upper body Core

My Thoughts

____

____

____

Eat to Live

It's time to continue learning how and what to eat. This is an important component of your weight loss, so pay close attention to all the tips and suggestions we give you to properly fuel your body and shed pounds.

DAY 15—**FOOD IS FUEL**

"Eat to live. Don't live to eat."
Socrates

A Word from Amy

After Rhett was diagnosed with autism, I went through all the stages of grief—denial, anger, bargaining, depression, and finally acceptance. During the day, I was the strong mother who pulled herself together to handle everything that needed to be done. Not only was I taking care of the household, but I was searching for cures, solutions, and therapies for Rhett. Surely there must be an answer, I thought, a healing, some way out.

At night, I was a wreck. I collapsed on the sofa in front of the TV and began to eat and eat and eat. I ate to deal with the events of the day. I ate through my grief. I ate to the point of numbness. I ate until I finally was able to fall asleep. When I finally surrendered to God and came to unconditionally accept Rhett as he was, I was still eating my way through the acceptance. I was shocked to find out I could no longer fit into even my largest clothes. Something was seriously wrong with my eating habits, and I knew it was time to change.

So many of us have an unhealthy relationship with food. We eat when we're happy and when we're depressed. We eat when we're bored and when we're anxious. We eat when we're stressed and when we want to celebrate. It's a sad truth, but many of us attach emotion to eating. But this is not how God wired us. We were created to eat to live, not live to eat.

There is nothing wrong with having a piece of cake or a slice of pizza in moderation. It's when we start gorging on the stuff out of some emotional need that we are headed for disaster. If you eat for pleasure because it tastes good, how good does it makes you feel afterward to see that pasta now sitting on your hips?

We had to learn that there were other pleasures in life besides eating. There's a whole nother world out there for you to enjoy and explore. So the next time you pick up your fork, remember why you are eating. You are eating to live.

Mini-Challenge of the Day

Apply the *wait technique.* When you want to eat foods that are not in your food plan for that day, be aware. *Wait.* Take a deep breath. Pray. Listen to your heart and ask, "Why do I want to eat this food right now? Am I hungry or bored or (fill in the blank)?" If you look deep inside, you will find the answer. You'll see that your desire for food doesn't have much to do with food at all. Use this technique over and over. It's hard in the beginning, but it will help you to slowly master your emotions instead of allowing your emotions to master you.

Tip of the Day

Phil and I make all our meals for the week on Sunday, and then store them in baggies and containers in the freezer. It saves a tremendous amount of time during the busy work week and keeps us more motivated to stick to our food plan.

Meal	Record Your Food & Water Intake for the Day	Calories
1		
2		
3		
4		
5		
	Total Calories	

Fitness Plan

Cardio activity: ____________________ Time: ________ Miles: ______

Intensity level (circle one): L M H

Strength training (circle): Lower body Upper body Core

My Thoughts

____

____

____

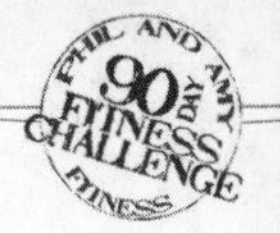

DAY 16—FOOD JOURNALING

"The more food records people kept, the more weight they lost. Those who kept daily food records lost twice as much weight as those who kept no records."

Jack Hollis, PhD, researcher at Kaiser Permanente Center for Health Research

A Note from Phil

Food journaling—keeping track of what you eat—is your secret weapon for weight loss. It's been proven that when people write down what they eat, they consume fewer calories. When you use a food journal, you know exactly what you are eating, when you are eating it, and where you are likely to overeat.

If you are allotted a specific number of calories per day, food journaling will help you determine how many calories you have eaten and how many calories you have left. This helped me a whole lot. It made me assess how many calories were in the foods I was eating and helped me to choose my foods wisely. (I use *The CalorieKing Calorie, Fat and Carbohydrate Counter* by Allan Borushek to help me keep track.)

From the first day on the ranch, we had to record our food intake in a food journal every day. Sometimes I would be so tired from working out that I'd try to avoid it like the plague. As the days went by I realized, however, how important it was to keep up this habit. We always kept our journal on the kitchen table and would write down the food we were eating as we ate.

The most important thing to keep in mind is to be honest about the food you are writing down. If you chew a piece of gum, write it down. If you eat two cheeseburgers, write it down. Never be afraid to face the truth that stares back at you through the food journal. You may also want to use this method to remind yourself to take your vitamins and keep track of how much water you drank that day. I also recommend jotting down your feelings. So much of your emotions are associated with food, especially in the beginning stages of weight loss. I am sure food journaling will help you as much as it has helped us.

Mini-Challenge of the Day

By now, you should have been writing in the food journal section in these devotions. If you haven't started, start *today* and commit to writing in your journal every day for thirty days. If you've already started, great job! Now go through the last two weeks of journal entries. Notice any habits that are forming. Do you indulge in late night snacks? Do you eat more on the weekends? Are you eating too much food that isn't prepared fresh? Are you not spreading your calories throughout the day? Pick one area and commit to changing it for the better.

Tip of the Day

Write as you go. We found if we wait until the end of the day to write down each item, it's easy to forget the details. To avoid this problem, get a portable journal (a small notebook or even a software program on your phone) you can take with you wherever you go.

Meal	Record Your Food & Water Intake for the Day	Calories
1		
2		
3		
4		
5		
	Total Calories	

Fitness Plan

Cardio activity: ______________________ Time: ________ Miles: ______

Intensity level (circle one): L M H

Strength training (circle): Lower body Upper body Core

My Thoughts

____

____

____

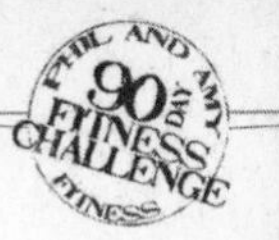

DAY 17—A DRINKING PROBLEM

"Up to 60 percent of the human body is water, the brain is composed of 70 percent water, and the lungs are nearly 90 percent water."

U.S. Department of the Interior

A Word from Amy

Many people have a drinking problem and I am not talking about being alcoholics. Their problem is that they are not drinking enough water. Water is so important that we literally can't live without it. In modern society we have substituted sodas and other drinks for God's drink of choice—good ol' H_2O.

Before being on *The Biggest Loser*, I rarely drank water. Once I started the health program on the ranch, I quickly saw the repercussions. Even though I was working out more than I ever had in my life, I didn't break a sweat for several days. The doctors were actually concerned about my health. My system was so clogged from all the processed foods and lack of water that my body was incapable of producing sweat. After a couple of weeks, my system normalized, but I learned an invaluable lesson about how vital water is to my health.

So how much water should you drink? Divide your weight in half and convert that number into ounces. That's how much water you should be drinking per day. So if you weigh 200 pounds, you would drink 100 ounces of water or 10 glasses that are 10 ounces each. This will ensure that you stay hydrated. You want the water to keep you hydrated but also flush out waste and toxins.

Another reason to drink water is to replace those soft drinks that can sabotage your weight-loss goals. Regular sodas are loaded with sugar and calories, but don't go buy a Diet Coke just yet. Diet sodas contain artificial sweeteners, which trigger your taste buds and make you think you are hungry. So diet sodas are as bad, if not worse, than regular ones. This is what we had to do to completely make the change. Drink water instead.

It is always a bad idea to drink your calories. Beware of how much juice, milk, and other liquids you drink because the calories add up in no time. Make sure you write down in your food journal what you drink as well as what you eat.

Mini-Challenge of the Day

If you don't have one yet, buy yourself a water bottle. Find one that doesn't leak from the cap and holds between sixteen and twenty ounces of liquid. If it's plastic, find one that is BPA-Free; it's a better type of plastic. The bottle should have a BPA-Free label on it, usually on the bottom.

Tip of the Day

Did you know that cravings come when you are dehydrated? If you don't drink enough water, you might think you are hungry when your body is actually crying out for something to drink. You never want to be without water for too long. You may want to keep a gallon or two of water in your car, just in case.

Meal	Record Your Food & Water Intake for the Day	Calories
1		
2		
3		
4		
5		
	Total Calories	

Fitness Plan

Cardio activity: ______________________ Time: ________ Miles: ______

Intensity level (circle one): L M H

Strength training (circle): Lower body Upper body Core

My Thoughts

____

____

____

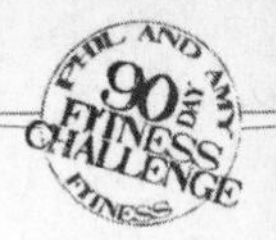

DAY 18—BAD WORDS

"Research has shown that even small amounts of processed food alter the chemical balance in our brain and cause negative mood swings along with noticeable dips in energy."

Marilu Henner

A Note from Phil

It's amazing how many bad words we use in our lives every day. I'm not talking about the colorful four-letter ones we say, but the ones we eat. Have you ever looked at the ingredients on a food label? Many of the words are impossible to pronounce, but more importantly I'm sure most of us don't even know what they are. Here are a few of the common "bad words" I'm talking about: *monosodium glutamate, partially hydrogenated oil, sodium nitrate, high fructose corn syrup, artificial flavoring, additives, preservatives,* and *antibiotics.* These are ingredients in our food that we should try our best to avoid.

A lot of companies add preservatives, different types of fat, and chemicals to make the food taste or look better, but our bodies are not meant to process all that junk. The FDA lists approximately 2800 food additives and about 3000 chemicals that are deliberately added to our food supply. Yikes.

Here is something to think about. Did you know that the FDA doesn't even make flavor companies disclose the ingredients of their additives as long as all the chemicals are considered by the agency to be Generally Regarded as Safe (GRAS)? I think it's interesting that the same chemicals with a slight variation can make something smell like a sweet dessert or a household product.

Our bodies are a living and breathing organism, not a chemical dumping ground.

And guess what? Your body actually craves fresh and natural foods. The more processed foods you eat, the less nutrients your body gets and metabolizes, leaving you still hungry. Not only that, but the chemicals in processed foods have been shown to be a contributing factor in low energy, mood swings, allergies, hyperactivity, asthma, depression, and even cancer.

Always remember that there is no substitute for fresh, natural, whole food. The more you learn to prepare foods yourself with natural ingredients, the better you will feel and the more your body will function at its optimum.

Mini-Challenge of the Day

Pick up two packaged foods that you would normally eat and read their food labels. If you don't know what some of the ingredients are, you probably shouldn't be eating it. Just toss those items right in the trash, but hold on to the label. For all the ingredients you are not familiar with, go to the Internet and research what they are. You will be surprised at what you are really eating. Some of you will even be shocked. Knowledge is power. Make reading food labels a part of your daily routine.

Tip of the Day

Remember the saying "Don't judge a book by its cover"? Well, use the same wise advice for food. When you buy bread, for example, read the label. All wheat breads look healthy, but looks can be deceiving. Look for the word *whole* on the label. Whole grain, whole wheat, and stone-ground whole wheat are winners.

Meal	Record Your Food & Water Intake for the Day	Calories
1		
2		
3		
4		
5		
	Total Calories	

Fitness Plan

Cardio activity: ____________________ Time: ________ Miles: ______

Intensity level (circle one): L M H

Strength training (circle): Lower body Upper body Core

My Thoughts

____

____

____

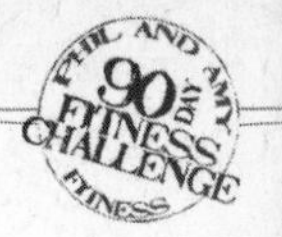

DAY 19—BE SURE TO EAT

"Obesity in the United States is a tremendous problem. And what we found, observing these otherwise healthy people, is that it's much better for people to spread their caloric intake out over multiple smaller meals throughout the day."

Yunsheng Ma, PhD, University of Maryland Medical System

A Word from Amy

As I write this, I am sitting in my office eating a Wasa cracker with some Laughing Cow cheese. Although I have crumbs all over my desk and computer keyboard, I am following one of the main rules of weight loss: eat between meals. I know we can all hear our mothers yelling at us that we're going to spoil our dinner if we do this, but (wince) they were wrong. You should eat every three to four hours.

Imagine your body is a car. It has to have gas every so many miles. In the same sense, our bodies have to have food throughout the day. Many people eat one huge meal and then starve the rest of the day. That's like throwing an entire pile of wood on a fire; it burns, but it burns out quickly. Others think they should eat three square meals a day. That's not a bad thing, but what's even better is eating a few small meals throughout the day. That's like throwing pieces of wood onto a fire as they're needed, making it burn longer.

Eating this way will help to keep your metabolism burning at a good rate for the whole day. Whatever number of calories you should be eating a day, try to break that up into six smaller meals. You'll soon find out that you won't feel hungry during the day.

But just as you wouldn't put sugar in your gas tank, you don't want to put food that's not good for you into your body. Before my weight-loss journey, my snacks came from vending machines. I ate all sorts of junk food—soda, chips, candy. I also thought that when I snacked, I was being bad. But snacking wasn't the problem. The problem was I was snacking on all the wrong foods. A good rule of thumb is to make sure your snacks have a good balance of protein, carbohydrates, and natural fat. (You can refer to some of our snacks and meals in appendix C.) This will keep your blood sugar level stabilized and keep those cravings to eat everything in the fridge from hitting you.

Here are some snacks we regularly eat:

- apple slices and almonds
- Wasa cracker and cheese or turkey
- yogurt with flaxseed
- tuna with mustard on a wheat cracker
- orange and pistachios
- carrots, broccoli, celery sticks with hummus
- blue corn chips and salsa
- granola or Kashi with almond milk
- small salad with salsa or mustard for dressing
- air-popped popcorn
- handful of mixed nuts
- rice cake with peanut butter
- banana and peanut butter

Mini-Challenge of the Day

Do not skip any meals! Even if you don't feel hungry, eat all your meals on your plan. The joke about how fat people don't ever miss a meal is a lie. Many people are fat because they miss meals all day and then pig out at night. I did exactly that and messed up my metabolism for a long time. What have you got to lose by eating more? Pounds!

Tip of the Day

Eat one to two apples a day to help regulate your blood sugar. Apples also help reduce your appetite and are a wonderful natural snack.

Meal	Record Your Food & Water Intake for the Day	Calories
1		
2		
3		
4		
5		
	Total Calories	

Fitness Plan

Cardio activity: ____________________ Time: ________ Miles: ______

Intensity level (circle one): L M H

Strength training (circle): Lower body Upper body Core

My Thoughts

____

____

____

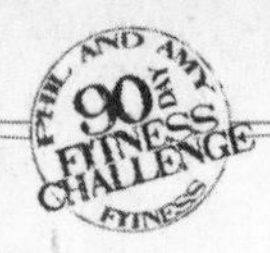

DAY 20—IT'S OK TO BE FRUITY

"An apple a day keeps the doctor away."

A Word from Amy

Where do fruits fit in our diet? Fruit is a wonderful source of vitamins, fiber, and antioxidants. Fruit is a carbohydrate and that is what gives us energy for workouts. It helps you feel full, it's delicious, and there are so many to choose from that you will never get bored.

We always try to mix a carb with a protein to keep our blood sugar stable. For example, when you are eating an apple or an orange, have some nuts or cheese with it. If you are having a yogurt, mix a little fruit such as peaches or berries in it. A little natural peanut or almond butter on a banana is my favorite snack.

As a general rule, nutritionists recommend two to four servings of fruit a day. Eat whole fruit, mix it in your oatmeal or cereal, or add it to protein shakes. A delicious way to get your fruit servings, especially in the summer, is to juice it. I'm not talking about the juice you buy in a container. I'm talking about using a juicing machine to extract the juice out of the fruit. Instead of buying a carton of orange juice, you can enjoy fresh orange juice for breakfast.

I had a friend tell me that she was able to control her craving for sweets by freezing grapes and eating them like candy while she watched TV. You can do the same thing with blueberries. I have also placed frozen strawberries in a blender to make a sorbet. You can do this with any frozen fruit. Here's one more idea. Peel a banana, stick a popsicle stick through the middle, freeze it, and you have a banana ice pop.

I recommend sticking with frozen or fresh fruit when you can. Canned fruit has too much sugar and has been through too much processing. Dried fruit and freeze-dried fruit, although delicious, are loaded with a higher concentrate of sugar. It's easier to overeat on these treats because they taste so sweet. Eating too much sugar could spike your blood sugar levels very fast and make you eat more. So stick with fresh fruit. It is nature's dessert and oh-so yummy.

Mini-Challenge of the Day

Think about how you can integrate two to four servings of fruit a day this week. Will you have a fruit snack in the afternoon? Will you make a piece of fruit part of your morning routine? Will you add a fruit for dessert or as a late night snack? The more regular you can make your routine, the easier it will be to keep it.

Tip of the Day

A fun and healthy snack is applesauce. Buy an organic brand, sprinkle a bit of cinnamon on it, and you have a delicious fruit snack with little to no preservatives. Cinnamon has been shown to help regulate insulin and blood sugar. It normalizes appetite and helps release fat reserves.

Meal	Record Your Food & Water Intake for the Day	Calories
1		
2		
3		
4		
5		
	Total Calories	

Fitness Plan

Cardio activity: ______________________ Time: ________ Miles: ______

Intensity level (circle one): L M H

Strength training (circle): Lower body Upper body Core

My Thoughts

____

____

____

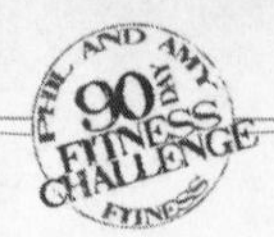

DAY 21—EATING HEALTHY WHEN EATING OUT

"Another good reducing exercise consists in placing both hands against the table edge and pushing back."

ROBERT QUILLEN

A Word from Amy

Restaurants. They are tough to face when you're focusing on weight loss. It's unrealistic to think you will never eat out. Not only is it convenient, it's a social activity. We meet friends over dinner. We close business deals over lunch. We celebrate anniversaries and birthday parties at restaurants. And what about when you travel or go on vacation? If you can't cook at home, you have no choice but to eat out.

Have no fear. No matter where you go out to eat, it is possible to eat properly. Restaurants are not evil places when you are in control of your choices and are equipped with knowledge to make your experience a healthy and enjoyable one. Here are a few of the tips we've learned along the way:

- Before you get to the restaurant, decide what you will eat. A lot of places have online menus and nutritional guides. If you know what you want before you go, you don't even have to look at a menu or be tempted by their daily specials.
- Don't eat the bread while you're waiting for your meal. Better yet, let your server know at the beginning that you don't want any bread. Out of sight, out of mind.
- Carry a bottle of salad dressing with you, something low fat, low calorie, and healthy.
- Make friends with your server. Your server can make sure that your food is prepared the way you want.
- Don't be shy. Ask your server if they can cook something that is not necessarily on the menu. You can also request to have your meal prepared without the added sauces, gravies, butters, oils, fats, and salt. Restaurant staffs are used to accommodating their customers, and you may be surprised by how they will want to make you happy.
- When in doubt, order grilled chicken with a side vegetable.

Almost every restaurant serves this. It may not be the most exciting thing on the menu, but it's a nutritional winner.

- Choose meats and fish that are grilled, broiled, or steamed.
- Avoid the wine. All alcohol turns to sugar in your system. If you are going to drink, then keep it within your calorie limit for the day.
- Skip the dessert and have a cup of black coffee instead.
- If we get big portions, I ask for a take-home container right up front. When the meal comes, I immediately put half of it in the container to take home with me.

Mini-Challenge of the Day

Pick two restaurants that you know you will be going to in the next few weeks. Find their online menus and nutritional information. Choose your meal today so when you go, you already know what you are going to eat. And stick to it.

Tip of the Day

I found that even if I ate well at a restaurant, I always felt a little bloated the next day. I figured out that restaurants generally use a lot of sodium in their cooking. Always ask for the no-salt or low-salt version, if possible.

Meal	Record Your Food & Water Intake for the Day	Calories
1		
2		
3		
4		
5		
	Total Calories	

Fitness Plan

Cardio activity: ____________________ Time: ________ Miles: ______

Intensity level (circle one): L M H

Strength training (circle): Lower body Upper body Core

My Thoughts

___

___

___

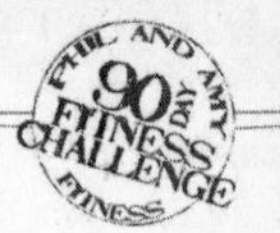

DAY 22—SUPERSIZE ME NOT

"Your eyes are always bigger than your stomach."
Confucius

A Note from Phil

In America, we believe that bigger is better. If you are buying a truck, why not go for the biggest truck on the market? If you can afford the bigger house, why not get the bigger house? We also have this idea that if we buy more of something, we are getting more value for our money. If you can supersize your meal and get twice the amount of french fries for only fifty cents more, why not? Well, that concept doesn't work when it comes to food and your health. The only value you receive by getting more bang for your buck is the added fat that's sitting on your waistline.

Our portion sizes are enormous in America, more than in any other country. It's probably one of the reasons our nation keeps getting fatter. In this lifestyle change that you have embarked on, it's important to learn about portion control. In the beginning of retraining your body to eat the right portions, you may feel hungry and think you're not eating enough food. But soon your stomach will adjust to the change and so will your eyes. You'll get used to eating a certain amount of food at each meal, and you'll be surprised how satisfied you feel.

Here are some tips to help you control your portions and lose weight:

- Here is a good rule of thumb for what one serving looks like:
  - A three-ounce serving of protein (chicken or fish) = deck of cards
  - One serving of complex carbohydrates/vegetables = two hands cupped together
  - One serving of whole grains (brown rice or oatmeal) = one hand cupped
- Get a kitchen scale and start weighing your food so you have an idea what a single serving size is. When I started this journey, I had to weigh everything until I got used to the right portion size.
- Put snacks in little baggies. Don't take a whole bag of nuts with you to the office. Prepack what you need for that day and take only that amount with you.

- If you have a lot of leftovers, freeze individual servings in separate containers. This way when you pull out something to eat, you don't have to reheat five servings and risk overeating. You can reheat only one serving at a time.
- When you go out to eat, if you can, order a kid's portion.

Mini-Challenge of the Day

Weigh or measure your food today. Make this a habit until you get more comfortable with portion sizes. If a serving size is one cup, don't just guess or pour it into a coffee mug. Coffee cups vary greatly in size. Get that measuring cup out and keep it handy. Keep your weight scale and measuring cups on the kitchen counter at all times.

Tip of the Day

Slow down while you eat. It takes fifteen minutes for your digestive system to tell your brain that you've had enough food. The best way to eat slower is to chew each mouthful thirty times. An added benefit is that the enzymes in your mouth help to break down the food, so it's easier to digest once it reaches your stomach. Take your time.

Meal	Record Your Food & Water Intake for the Day	Calories
1		
2		
3		
4		
5		
	Total Calories	

Fitness Plan

Cardio activity: ______________________ Time: ________ Miles: ______

Intensity level (circle one): L M H

Strength training (circle): Lower body Upper body Core

My Thoughts

___

___

___

DAY 23—**SHAKE THE SALT**

"A spoon of salt in a glass of water makes the water undrinkable. A spoon of salt in a lake is almost unnoticed."
BUDDHA

A Note from Phil

Monitoring salt intake is one of the most important things we've learned through our weight-loss process. Excess sodium is unhealthy for your heart, causes water retention, and increases blood pressure. The American Heart Association recommends no more than 2400 milligrams of sodium per day. It's said that the average American consumes 4000 milligrams per day. We try to keep our sodium intake under 1500 milligrams.

The next time you read a food label, take a look at the sodium content. The first time I checked a can of soup, which I thought was healthy, I saw it contained 1000 milligrams of sodium. That little can was over half my sodium limit for the day. You'll be surprised at how much sodium processed foods have, which is one reason why we suggest you avoid processed foods altogether. Also, monitor how often you go out to eat. As we've said before, most restaurants are liberal with how much salt they use in their cooking.

I know what many of you are thinking. *If I don't use salt, everything is going to taste bland.* That's just not true. When you dump the salt habit, you actually begin to taste the food you are eating. Everything has a flavor. Learn to appreciate the flavors and textures of foods without salt.

Amy and I have learned to spice up the flavor of food with salt alternatives. They are better than salt because they enhance rather than mask the flavor of foods. Here are some alternatives you might want to try:

- salt substitute (potassium)
- lemon/lime
- chili/cayenne pepper
- herbs such as basil, thyme, rosemary (fresh and dried)
- onions and garlic
- spices such as cilantro, curry, oregano, and pepper
- Mrs. Dash premixed, salt-free seasoning (it's one of our favorites)

Here are some other tips to help you reduce the sodium in your diet:

- Cook with low-sodium chicken broth.
- Don't salt your pasta or rice water.
- Rinse canned fish and vegetables to remove some of the salt.

Mini-Challenge of the Day

Take the salt out of your diet. Remove all saltshakers and salt in your house. If you are not doing this already, eat all your foods unsalted. Experience the true flavor and texture of food. This is the first step in relearning what foods really taste like.

Tip of the Day

Try to avoid smoked meats and processed meats such as bologna, hot dogs, and salami. They are usually high in fat and sodium. They also contain nitrates that have been linked to different cancers. If you do need to choose a lunch meat, make a better choice by choosing a low-sodium brand.

Meal	Record Your Food & Water Intake for the Day	Calories
1		
2		
3		
4		
5		
	Total Calories	

Fitness Plan

Cardio activity: ______________________ Time: ________ Miles: ______

Intensity level (circle one): L M H

Strength training (circle): Lower body Upper body Core

My Thoughts

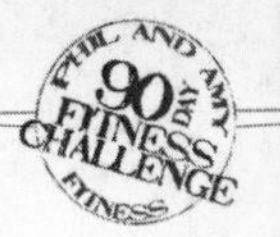

DAY 24—HOPE FLOATS

"The best sources of fiber come from food. Taking a supplement or multiple vitamin can't replace the damage of a poor diet."

LINDA VON HORN, PHD, RD

A Note from Phil

I've got a fun subject for you. How many times a day do you have a bowel movement? If you aren't going on average one to three times a day, then chances are you don't have enough fiber in your diet.

We are supposed to have about twenty-five to thirty grams of fiber in our diet every day. Fiber is like the Drano for our intestines; it keeps our pipes clean. Fiber is also excellent for weight control. It expands in your stomach so it keeps you feeling full. The fuller you feel, the less hungry you will be. How do you know if you are getting enough fiber in your diet? Do the quick "float test." Next time you have a bowel movement, take a look. If your stool floats, then you are getting adequate fiber in your diet. If it sinks like the Titanic, then Houston, we might have a fiber problem.

Here are some easy ways to get your fiber. The easiest is buying fiber supplements and putting them in shakes, but Amy and I always like to get our nutrients naturally. Look for high-fiber breakfast cereals. If you eat a bowl in the morning, you are off to a good start. We eat Kashi or Fiber One because these cereals have twelve grams of fiber per serving. Apples, oranges, carrots, broccoli, whole grain breads and pastas, kidney beans, and garbanzo beans are a few more examples of higher-fiber foods. Read the food labels to see how much fiber you are getting per serving. Some whole wheat breads have only two grams of fiber where others have much more. If you have to choose between similar products, always buy the one with higher fiber. One last note, fruit and vegetable juices have little or no fiber since the juicing process removes the bulk. So don't drink your veggies; eat them instead.

Mini-Challenge of the Day

How does fiber fit into your new lifestyle today? First, do the float test. Second, how many times a day are you having bowel movements? Lastly, pick two ways you will introduce more fiber in your diet naturally. Make this a habit and start today.

Tip of the Day

The greener the lettuce, the more nutrients it has. Iceberg lettuce has little nutritional value. The color of this leafy green is also very light. Change your lettuces to the ones that are darker green such as romaine lettuce, spinach, or escarole.

Meal	Record Your Food & Water Intake for the Day	Calories
1		
2		
3		
4		
5		
	Total Calories	

Fitness Plan

Cardio activity: ____________________ Time: ________ Miles: ______

Intensity level (circle one): L M H

Strength training (circle): Lower body Upper body Core

My Thoughts

____

____

____

DAY 25—SHEDDING POUNDS AND HAVING FUN

"The doors we open and close each day decide the lives we live."
FLORA WHITTEMORE

What an inspiration April has been! Before she joined the "Challenge," she was on a diet and had already lost a few pounds. What she needed, however, was a jumpstart as her weight loss was slowing down and she was getting bored. As April continued on with the "Challenge," the pounds came right off. Here is her story.

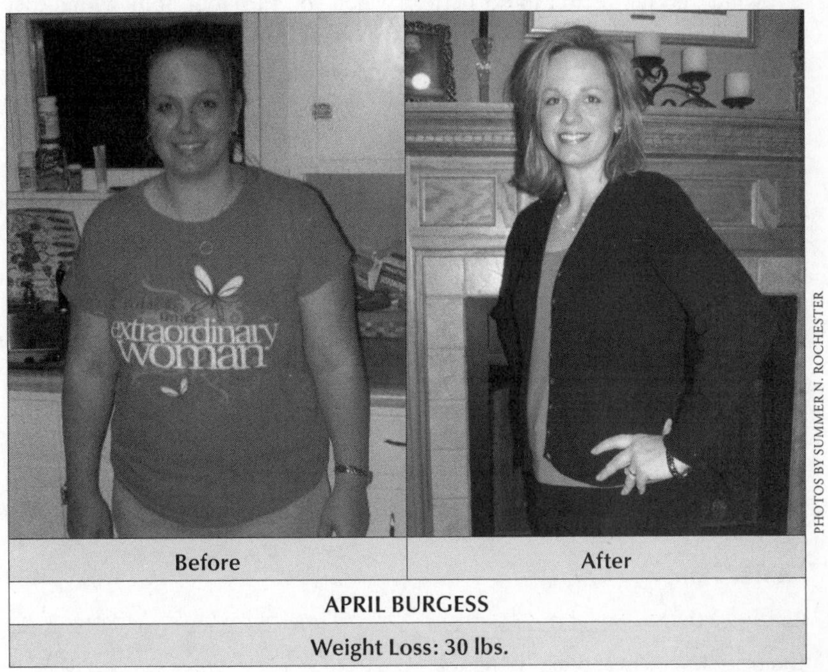

Before	After
APRIL BURGESS	
Weight Loss: 30 lbs.	

PHOTOS BY SUMMER N. ROCHESTER

"My name is April Burgess. I joined the '90-Day Challenge' weighing 204 pounds, but originally started losing weight when I weighed 216 pounds. I took the 'Challenge' as the fire I needed to spring my rear into gear. I got serious about working out and controlling my portion sizes, and looking to other things for pleasure instead of food. I am currently at 176 pounds and plan to lose more. I have lost ten inches off my waist.

"I get frequent compliments on my new body and shopping is so much more fun. But the best thing in losing all this weight is knowing that I am accomplishing goals I have set. No more looking back, being no better off than I was, and wishing that I had stuck to a diet."

Mini-Challenge of the Day

You've heard the quote from Jesus, "It is more blessed to give than to receive." Today I want you to encourage someone who needs it. Maybe you know a friend who is sick, has relationship problems, or just feels blue. Pick up the phone and brighten their day with your positive and life-affirming words.

Tip of the Day

Want another reason to eat better? When you fuel your body with a diet high in fruits and vegetables, your skin will become noticeably smoother. Natural foods have tons of antioxidants that help protect the skin from stress and environmental damage.

Meal	Record Your Food & Water Intake for the Day	Calories
1		
2		
3		
4		
5		
	Total Calories	

Fitness Plan

Cardio activity: ____________________ Time: ________ Miles: ______

Intensity level (circle one): L M H

Strength training (circle): Lower body Upper body Core

My Thoughts

____

____

____

Activate Your Body

Did you know that you're already an athlete? Are you surprised? We'll show you what we mean in this section. You'll also learn that working out doesn't just mean going to the gym. You'll never look at exercise the same way again. You'll also be glad to know that rest (yeah!) is just as important as training.

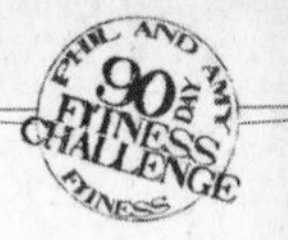

DAY 26—I AM AN ATHLETE

"The more I talk to athletes, the more convinced I become that the method of training is relatively unimportant. There are many ways to the top, and the training method you choose is just the one that suits you best. No, the important thing is the attitude of the athlete, the desire to get to the top."

Herb Elliott

A Note from Phil

When Amy and I started our own challenge, you could count on both hands how many times we had been in a gym in our entire lives. My athletic background was minimal compared to the average man my age. Plus, I was carrying an extra 150 pounds on my frame. For sure, I could not be classified as athletic.

While we were at the ranch, our trainers always referred to us as athletes. Every time I heard that description, I laughed. Surely they were joking. I thought, *They don't know anything about me. I am* not *an athlete.* If I ever said something to that effect out loud, our doctors and trainers would stop me and say, "Oh yes you are." They explained that the level and length of training we were going through was comparable to that of an Olympian. That about blew me away. We were also reminded that the extra weight we were all lugging around made our workouts even more challenging.

Through that experience, I realized that my life was similar to someone playing a professional sport or running a race. It was a competition. Most of the time I was competing only against myself, but I was competing nonetheless. I started believing that, yes, I was an athlete. I started viewing myself differently. I felt strong and empowered. Motivated and determined. This is who I really am.

When I thought of myself as an athlete, my mindset changed. Every step and every calorie mattered. My finish line was losing weight and being healthy. It was a competition for my life, and I was going to win! Take a look at yourself. How do you view yourself? Do you believe an athlete is hidden inside of you? I can tell you there is. Now own that truth and let the competition begin.

Mini-Challenge of the Day

Think back to your high school or college days. Did you participate in sports? If so, what kind of mentality did you have as an athlete? How did you motivate yourself to push harder through the times you wanted to give up? If you didn't play a sport, think about an area in your life where you are driven. How are you fueled to do your best by competition? Use these thoughts to motivate you to assume the mindset of an athlete—powerful, strong, and able.

Tip of the Day

Watch your coffee intake. Caffeine is a stimulant and releases the stress hormone cortisol. Many experts believe that increased levels of cortisol lead to stronger cravings for fat and carbohydrates and cause the body to store fat in the abdomen. However, if you drink a cup before you exercise, it will give you a better performance boost. Limit yourself to one or two cups per day and preferably thirty minutes before you exercise.

Meal	Record Your Food & Water Intake for the Day	Calories
1		
2		
3		
4		
5		
	Total Calories	

Fitness Plan

Cardio activity: ____________________ Time: ________ Miles: ______

Intensity level (circle one): L M H

Strength training (circle): Lower body Upper body Core

My Thoughts

____

____

____

DAY 27—WHAT ABOUT WEIGHTS?

"A strong body makes the mind strong."
Thomas Jefferson

A Word from Amy

People frequently complain to me that their weight loss has slowed or stopped entirely. I always ask them the obvious questions. Are you drinking enough water? Are you watching your calories? Are you eating small meals every four hours? Are you balancing proteins, carbohydrates, and healthy fat with every meal and snack? Are you doing your cardio consistently? If the answer to all of these questions is yes, then I ask next if they are doing their weight training. Most of the time I get strange looks, especially from women. The perception is that lifting weights makes you big and bulky. I thought the same thing until I found out that just isn't true.

When I was on the ranch, my trainer, Bob Harper, told me I needed to lift weights because muscle burns fat. If you work on building muscle, you will burn more calories throughout the day. Bob had me do lots of weight training with my legs because, he advised, our legs contain some of the largest muscles in the entire body. Also, muscle weighs more than fat but takes up less room. If you incorporate weight training along with cardio exercise and maintain your diet plan, you might weigh the same but your clothes will be looser.

Here's another bonus to weight training. Well-toned muscles help your skin not to look as saggy. I consulted a plastic surgeon after the show because I was concerned about the excess skin around my midsection. The doctor said that both my husband and I looked better than anyone he had ever seen who had lost the amount of weight that we had. He attributed it to the weight training we had done.

So get out there and start pumping. Don't be scared, ladies, you won't end up looking like the Incredible Hulk. I promise you!

Mini-Challenge of the Day

Incorporate weight training into your exercise routine at least two days a week. Buy some hand weights and strength training DVDs and do your routine at home. Or join a gym and hire a personal trainer to show you how to use the machines and maximize your time. No matter how you do it, it's time to start weight training today.

Tip of the Day

Remember the saying "Strong body, strong mind" next time you go to the gym. Pick up those weights and give it your all. You might feel sore the next day and it might take your body a few weeks to get used to lifting, but soon you will notice that your mind is clearer and you feel stronger. You may think you are only conditioning your body, but you are also changing your mindset.

Meal	Record Your Food & Water Intake for the Day	Calories
1		
2		
3		
4		
5		
	Total Calories	

Fitness Plan

Cardio activity: ______________________ Time: ________ Miles: ______

Intensity level (circle one): L M H

Strength training (circle): Lower body Upper body Core

My Thoughts

____

____

____

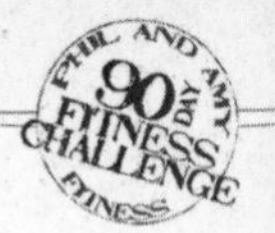

DAY 28—LET'S GET MOVING

"Those who think they have not time for bodily exercise will sooner or later have to find time for illness."
Edward Stanley

A Word from Amy

So many people tell me they have no time for exercise. We all know you have to make time. It was easy being on the ranch and having nothing to do but exercise. But when Phil and I came back to the real world and our many responsibilities, we had to intentionally clear out our schedules for exercise. We still schedule in our workouts because we understand that maintaining a healthy lifestyle requires consistent workouts.

We have also learned to stay active as much as we can and not only when we are at the gym. For instance, if I have to miss a workout because I have to clean the house for a holiday party, I don't get upset. I turn housecleaning into exercise. I jog up the stairs. When I dust, I exaggerate my movements and stretch up and down. When I vacuum, I swing my hips and move faster. Movement is exercise—don't forget that.

I never want to hear you say, "I don't have time to exercise." You do have time, you just have to schedule it or be creative as to how you get it. Any movement you do besides sitting on the couch and watching TV burns calories. Here are some examples that you might consider that will help you to both stay in shape and get your chores done around the house.

- Raking leaves. This causes you to use your arms and back. It is great cardio, especially when you bag the leaves and load them onto a truck or take them out to your curb.
- Cleaning out closets. This always makes me feel great. It involves heavy lifting, which can be great for your arms and legs. You also feel so good when you get rid of or donate stuff you don't need.
- Vacuuming, mopping, and sweeping the house = Cardio. The more floor, the more calories.
- Playing with your kids. Get excited! Run around the house with them. Play in the yard. That's a workout.
- Pruning trees. I did this a couple of weeks ago, and I was sore all over my body the next day so I know this is a great workout.

Mini-Challenge of the Day

List three ways you can incorporate movement into your daily routine. You can use some of the examples I gave, but also think of some others. For instance, think about what can you do if you work in an office during the day? How can you be active there?

____

____

____

Tip of the Day

Oatmeal really packs a punch. It is a slow-burning complex carbohydrate. It prolongs the feeling of fullness and prevents your blood sugar from rising too much. The soluble fiber in oatmeal fills you while lowering cholesterol. Did you know that oatmeal is one of the few foods rich in silicon? Silicon is a mineral responsible for building beautiful skin, hair, bones, and teeth. Beware of the prepackaged oatmeal that has added sugars. Use the slow-cooked or steel-cut kind and add some nuts, fruit, or raisins and your favorite natural sweetener.

Meal	Record Your Food & Water Intake for the Day	Calories
1		
2		
3		
4		
5		
	Total Calories	

Fitness Plan

Cardio activity: ______________ Time: ________ Miles: ______

Intensity level (circle one): L M H

Strength training (circle): Lower body Upper body Core

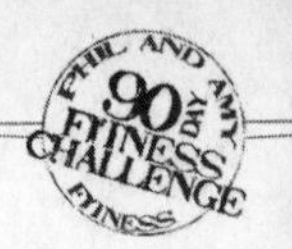

My Thoughts

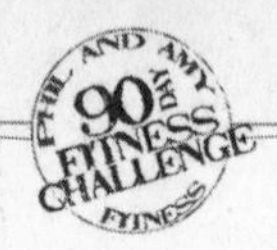

DAY 29—AMP IT UP

"If you want more, you have to require more from yourself."
Dr. Phil McGraw

A Word from Amy

I challenge you to amp up your fitness intensity. Walking is awesome in the beginning of your health journey, but when your body gets used it, you may need to kick your routine up a notch.

One way to do this, and to see some tremendous results, is by interval training. My trainer encouraged me to get my heart rate up really high for one minute and then bring it back down for a minute. I repeated this cycle for about an hour. You can do the same thing with almost any activity, such as walking outside or on a treadmill, cycling, or running up stairs and walking down. Group classes are also great for forcing you to stay at a certain level of intensity for a period of time.

We have to push ourselves to keep going to a higher level of strength and fitness. If you think you can do more, then do more. Work a little harder or extend your workout time a little longer. We always have to be switching things up on our bodies. When our body gets used to something, it will plateau and hold on to weight.

This is true with our diet too. If we eat the same amount of calories every day, then our bodies will say, "Hmm, I have this plan figured out. I am comfortable staying at this weight." To counteract this, I try to eat a different amount of calories every day. One day I'll eat 1200 calories, the next day 1400 calories, the next day 1600 calories. I keep my body guessing so it shocks my system and keeps me from the dreaded plateau.

Don't do the same routine day after day, week after week. Change up your workout habits every so often. Take a yoga class instead of a cycle class. Swim instead of run. Work out for an hour instead of thirty minutes. If you do this, your body will start changing sooner than you think. Go ahead, amp it up! I know you can do it.

Mini-Challenge of the Day

Challenge yourself today to extend your workout a little longer. Exercise for fifteen minutes more at a higher intensity or try walking farther than you did yesterday. You'll feel the difference.

Tip of the Day

If I find that my weight has reached a plateau, I will have a high calorie day—up to 2000 calories or more—but still eat healthy and nutritious foods. Then I'll drop my calories the next day to about 1200. This helps to shock my body into fat-burning mode again.

Meal	Record Your Food & Water Intake for the Day	Calories
1		
2		
3		
4		
5		
	Total Calories	

Fitness Plan

Cardio activity: ____________________ Time: ________ Miles: ______

Intensity level (circle one): L M H

Strength training (circle): Lower body Upper body Core

My Thoughts

____

____

____

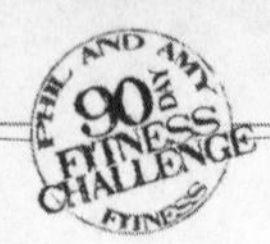

DAY 30—**MIX UP THE CARDIO**

"Variety is the spice of life."
William Cowper, English poet

A Word from Amy

If you've been exercising most days of the week, you should have a little more stamina now than you did when you started. That's great! Now let's take it a step further. We already talked about pushing yourself to the next level with intensity and interval training. Now it's time to start pushing yourself with variety.

Exercise is a lifestyle. For Phil and me, it wasn't about exercising just for the contest. We knew we had to make exercise a part of our lives forever. So it was important to think of new ways to spice up our fitness regimen to keep things interesting and motivating. You need to do the same thing.

You may already be bored to death of walking outside or on the treadmill. On the ranch, we walked for hours each day on the treadmill and around the campus. When I got home, I felt as if I had been brainwashed into some kind of "walking cult" because I was afraid if I wasn't walking I wasn't doing the right thing. One day, my sister-in-law encouraged me to go with her to a body combat class. I am not the most coordinated person in the world, so it took a little coaxing.

The first time I went, I stayed five minutes and then literally ran back to my safe little treadmill. The next day, I stood outside the class and watched. It looked as if the people in there were having fun punching and kicking. I needed to get some aggression out and decided to give it another try. Surprisingly, I was able to hang in there without accidentally kicking someone in the face. That class quickly became one of my favorite cardio workouts, and I went at least three times a week for a while. Each class was a little different than the last, so I always stayed interested.

I encourage you to try new things. Don't think that all you can do for exercise is walk. While it is convenient and you don't need to join a gym to do it, it will get boring after a while. The last thing you want to be is bored when you work out because you will eventually stop working out. Don't worry. There are tons of cardio options to choose from. You may not be able to start out doing some of them, but as you build up your strength and endurance, you can try the more challenging activities. Here is a list of ideas:

- Elliptical machine
- Swimming or water aerobics

- Step aerobics
- Tae Bo or kick boxing
- Spinning
- Yoga
- Exercise videos
- Dancing
- Rowing machine
- Racquetball
- Basketball
- Tennis
- Baseball/softball
- Boxing
- Stair climber
- Hiking
- Biking

Mini-Challenge of the Day

For every phone call you get today, do ten pushups after you hang up.

Tip of the Day

A great snack is five to ten unsalted almonds with an apple. The apple is nutritious and gives you energy, and the almonds are a healthy natural fat and help to slow down the release of sugar into your system.

Meal	Record Your Food & Water Intake for the Day	Calories
1		
2		
3		
4		
5		
	Total Calories	

Fitness Plan

Cardio activity: ______________________ Time: ________ Miles: ______

Intensity level (circle one): L M H

Strength training (circle): Lower body Upper body Core

My Thoughts

____

____

____

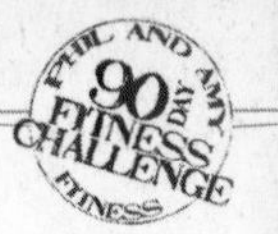

DAY 31—JUST A DAY IN THE PARK

"Man cannot discover new oceans unless he has the courage to lose sight of the shore."
André Gide

A Note from Phil

Like you, we have a busy lifestyle. Recently we took a day to reflect and have a little fun with the family. We got up at our normal time and went to the gym to work out. Then we came home, loaded up the kids, and drove to Furman University and had a picnic by the lake.

Our family laughed and chatted as we shared a healthy lunch, and then we took a stroll around the campus through the various lush gardens. I said to them, "Hey, if Mommy and Daddy hadn't lost this weight and gotten healthy, do you think we would have ever done this?" Our kids were quick to respond. "No way! We would've probably just driven around and bought some fast food for the picnic."

We then took the kids to the zoo and the playground. As we were walking around and playing with one another, I noticed how much more active our kids were getting. They were following our example. Later that night after dinner, we took them swimming at the community pool. It was a full day of fresh air, healthy food, exciting and calorie-burning activities, and beautiful time spent with the family.

Getting active is much more fun than not being active. Finding new ways to be active is like uncharted territory just waiting for you to explore. We are doing so many new things compared to when we lived a sedentary life. We've explored the parks in our town and have taken the kids hiking.

I encourage you to think about how making small changes today can result in a fully active lifestyle where you will not only be getting fit, but you will also be having fun. Think about the beautiful days you can enjoy with your loved ones hiking, running, and swimming. If you're not physically ready to do those things quite yet, keep working the "Challenge." You'll get there soon enough.

Mini-Challenge of the Day

Plan an outing with your family this week. Do something outdoors and make it fun and active.

Tip of the Day

Lots of people use food and snacks to break up their work routine, especially if they work in an office. Be careful. Don't let your work environment sabotage your meal plan. If you stick to your meal plan, you will be less hungry. If you start skipping meals because you are too busy, all of a sudden you'll find yourself reaching for the cake in the office kitchen or heading down to the vending machine.

Meal	Record Your Food & Water Intake for the Day	Calories
1		
2		
3		
4		
5		
	Total Calories	

Fitness Plan

Cardio activity: ____________________ Time: ________ Miles: _____

Intensity level (circle one): L M H

Strength training (circle): Lower body Upper body Core

My Thoughts

____

____

____

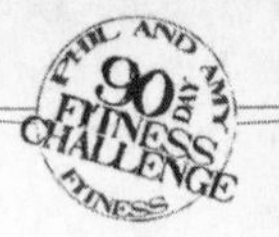

DAY 32—MAKE TIME TO RECOVER

"Rest when you're weary.
Refresh and renew yourself, your body,
your mind, your spirit. Then get back to work."
Ralph Marston

A Word from Amy

One of the important things to remember as you journey through this fitness challenge is to rest. If you're like me, this area is easy to neglect. Just ask anyone who knows me well. My mother once told me that when I was a little girl, putting me down for a nap was a nightmare because I always wanted to be where the action was. That part of me is still alive and kicking today. I like to be on the move, in the thick of things, doing and going nonstop.

Phil makes fun of me on the days I emotionally break down. He's not being mean, he just knows me well. In the middle of me sobbing about the world falling apart, he smiles at me and gently asks, "Amy, how many hours of sleep did you have last night? And the night before? And the night before that?" It's as if a lightbulb turns on in my head. I realize my problem is not that I'm an emotional wreck, I'm just tired. It's that plain and simple.

Our bodies need rest for several reasons. Rest keeps our hormones balanced and helps our metabolism to stay active. If we don't allow our bodies to rest, they will repay us by hanging on to unwanted weight. Rest gives you the energy you need for your workouts. Rest gives your body recovery time to recharge and build muscle. Rest keeps you emotionally stable. Rest helps keep your eating habits in check. Rest is good.

When we were on the ranch, Jillian Michaels would sometimes send people out of the gym and tell them to go and take a nap. She's one of the top fitness trainers in the country, so she must really believe in the principle of recovery to tell someone to take a break. She knows that successful weight loss requires the proper amount of rest.

One more thing. You know what happens if you're training and don't get proper rest? Your body is more apt to get injured because it is tired. Not only that, but overtraining without recovery can make you feel depressed and may even decrease your performance so your workouts fall below par. I've noticed many times when I take a day off and give my body a break, my next workouts are amazing. I feel more powerful, strong, and energized.

So to all of you type-A personalities like me who think that you can survive with limited sleep...think again. You must get proper rest.

Mini-Challenge of the Day

Have you recently felt tired or sluggish? Are you getting enough sleep? Are you training too hard? Analyze your exercise and rest habits in the last week. See if there is a balance. If there is, great! You are on the right track. If not, I give you permission to take a nap today or get eight hours of sleep every night this week.

Tip of the Day

I suggest you weigh in the same time every week and no more than once a week. It should be the first thing you do in the morning after you use the bathroom. I also suggest measuring your body periodically with a tape measure. Using the scale as your only guide can be misleading; losing inches tells part of the story too.

Meal	Record Your Food & Water Intake for the Day	Calories
1		
2		
3		
4		
5		
	Total Calories	

Fitness Plan

Cardio activity: ____________________ Time: ________ Miles: ______

Intensity level (circle one): L M H

Strength training (circle): Lower body Upper body Core

My Thoughts

____

____

____

DAY 33—FRIENDS STICK TOGETHER

"Birds of a feather flock together."
PROVERB

You can't meet April without loving her. She and her friend Thom joined the "90-Day Fitness Challenge" together. Watching those two on their journey reminded us of how important support is when you're trying to lose weight and better your health. Together these two people shed pounds and gained health. Read April's story.

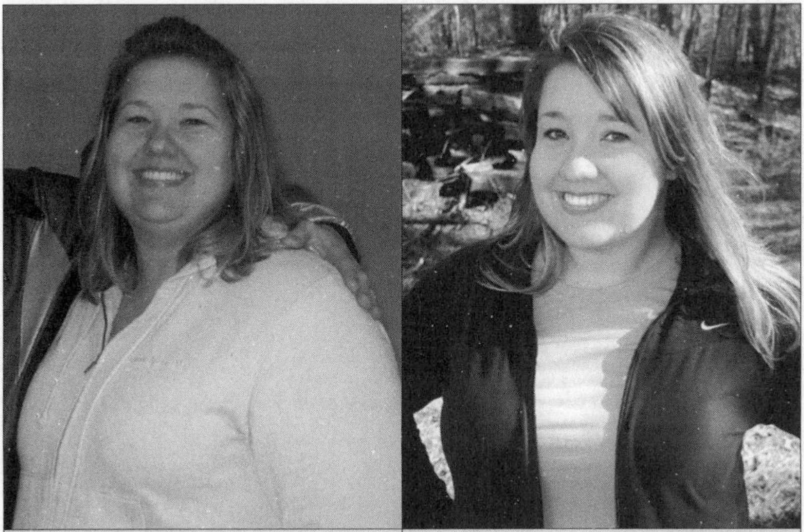

PHOTO BY MARY MCQUAID

PHOTO BY LAUREN N. HIGHSMITH

Before	After
APRIL GRAY	
Weight Loss: 60 lbs.	

"My best friend, Thom, challenged me to change my life by joining the '90-Day Fitness Challenge.' I'm not naturally a competitive person, but my determination to lose weight fueled my passion to change my life. Thom and I joined the 'Challenge' with his aunt and her friend. For the first time, I felt empowered to speak openly of my weight struggle, to share my experiences with loving friends, and to take public and strong steps toward a long-lasting change.

Truthfully, I would never have joined without Thom's encouragement and support. He encourages and speaks the truth, even when it's really hard to hear.

"All four of us track our running mileage, discuss our meals, celebrate 'floaters,' and guzzle water together. When we're tempted to cheat, we compromise in a healthful way by splitting meals or eating half. I always thought that it would be humiliating to share these struggles with someone, but doing so has made me a stronger person. I swallowed my shame and let myself be encouraged and supported by loving friends. We laugh, sweat, grunt, and encourage each other throughout the week. What a huge loss it would have been to let my fat-fear keep me from this amazing group of people.

"This year has been transformational. I've toned up, found muscles that have been buried for years, and gained peace, confidence, and energy through exercise. My after picture was taken on a hike that I would have never been able to do at my previous weight. It was a one-hour vertical climb just to get to the waterfall. Amy and Phil got me started and helped me change my life."

Mini-Challenge of the Day

Call up a friend and ask for his or her favorite healthy recipe that's easy to make. Make that dish today or at least buy the ingredients and make it this weekend. You will have both connected with a friend and discovered a new, good-for-you recipe.

Tip of the Day

Never shop casually up and down every aisle in the supermarket. This is dangerous as most of the unhealthy processed and packaged foods are located in the aisles. Instead, shop the perimeter of the store. This is where the healthiest foods are, such as fruits, vegetables, dairy, and protein.

Meal	Record Your Food & Water Intake for the Day	Calories
1		
2		
3		
4		
5		
	Total Calories	

Fitness Plan

Cardio activity: ____________________ Time: ________ Miles: ______

Intensity level (circle one): L M H

Strength training (circle): Lower body Upper body Core

My Thoughts

____

____

____

Mental Strategies: Creating New Mindsets

Changing your mindset is just as important as changing your body. After reading this challenge section, you will be equipped with strategies to think like the winner that you are. Learn how to be in charge of your mind, the importance of having a positive attitude, and making the commitment to never give up. You'll also become a pro at making mini-goals and having the flexibility to deal with change.

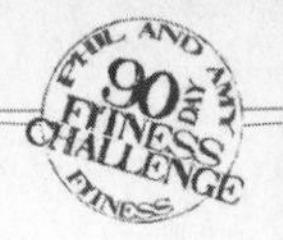

DAY 34—WHAT'S YOUR STRATEGY?

"Imagination is more important than knowledge. For while knowledge defines all we currently know and understand, imagination points to all we might yet discover and create."

Albert Einstein

A Word from Amy

We have said many times that the body follows the mind. The thoughts you think and the beliefs you have will determine the direction your life is headed. What does this mean when it comes to fitness? It means we need to have some mental strategies in place to keep us on the path toward a healthier life. Here are a few tips that have helped us on our journey.

1. Imagine. Imagine what your life will be like when you reach your goals. What will you look like? What will it feel like to buy clothes in a smaller size? What will it feel like to be able to run a race? Imagine with the confidence that those things will come to pass.

2. Tell yourself it's your idea. One thing I do when I'm lying in bed fighting with myself about getting up to work out is to tell myself how much I love exercise. Sometimes just telling yourself that you love something makes it easier to do. You can actually convince yourself that something is fun even when it's hard. Tell yourself you love veggies. Tell yourself you love running. Tell yourself you love preparing your own healthy meals. Train your mind to do what's right by telling yourself how much you like doing it. Soon, I promise you, you really *will* like doing them.

3. Watch your mouth. Be aware of the negative words that come out of your mouth. Don't say "I have to go to the gym." Say "I get to go the gym." Don't tell yourself all the reasons why you "can't" exercise or eat well. Tell yourself that you "are able" to do all these things. When I was on the show, hearing certain teammates talking negatively easily brought me down. I learned, however, to talk to myself in a positive way and ignore that negative speak.

4. Remember your blessings. So many people are less fortunate than we are. There are men and women all over the world who are so sick they are unable to focus on their health. Many are incapable of exercising. When I feel as though I can't run any farther during my workouts, I think of all the people without legs who could only dream of running. It's a great reality check for me and makes me grateful for everything I have—the good and even the bad.

When the going gets tough, it's time to put these strategies into action. Let them fuel you to keep going when your mind is telling you otherwise.

Mini-Challenge of the Day

I gave you four ways to push through the challenges that are inevitable in your weight-loss journey. Perhaps by now you have created some of your own. If not, now is the right time. In the space below, create a three-step battle plan for conquering the difficult times in the journey. Perhaps you might pray or go to a support group or read some Scripture. Whatever your strategy for keeping your mind in check, practice it regularly so it becomes second nature.

____

____

____

Tip of the Day

Eat before you go to parties. If you go to an event on an empty stomach, you will be tempted to eat all the finger foods that are typically high in fat and sugar. Load up on fruits and veggies before you go so you won't be hungry. At the party, have a few tastes of the food and avoid the rest. You won't feel deprived and you won't overeat.

Meal	Record Your Food & Water Intake for the Day	Calories
1		
2		
3		
4		
5		
	Total Calories	

Fitness Plan

Cardio activity: ____________________ Time: ________ Miles: ______

Intensity level (circle one): L M H

Strength training (circle): Lower body Upper body Core

My Thoughts

___

___

___

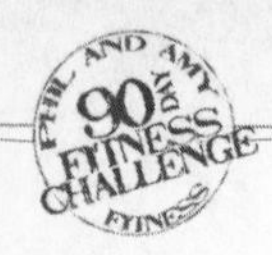

DAY 35—**YOUR TRUTH OR *THE* TRUTH**

"A wise man changes his mind, a fool never."
Spanish Proverb

A Note from Phil

One of the biggest obstacles that you will face in this "Challenge" (if you haven't figured it out already) is your mind. Think back to when you started this journey. Your mentality has probably changed since then in a positive way, especially as your overall health habits changed for the better. As you continue to lose weight, this process will bring up so many different thoughts and feelings. Some are good and others are not. Some of the "old you" thinking may pop up out of nowhere and hinder your progress. I know. It happened to me.

One thing I battled for years was that I didn't finish what I started. This character trait haunted me. Somewhere during my childhood, someone told me I was a quitter. Instead of defending myself, I chose to believe that negative statement. I owned it and made it a part of me well into adulthood. I actually lived out that thought day to day and replayed it in my mind without even questioning it. But was it true? Was I really a quitter?

While I did give up once in a while on projects, the fact was this negative statement was not *the* truth. I had, however, allowed it to become my truth. I remember one day on the ranch when we were all exercising real hard. As I looked around me, I saw most of my peers struggling with their workouts. The old thought pattern suddenly came to me, *Well, I guess it's time to quit.* But just before I made the choice to entertain the old me, I thought instead, *No, I am strong! I am going to keep going. I am not going to quit.* I made the decision right there to finish my workouts that time and every time.

Changing my mindset didn't happen overnight. I cannot tell you how many times I was working out and would be so exhausted I was tempted to quit. I had to tell myself over and over, *No! The new Phil finishes what he starts. The new Phil doesn't give up. The new Phil will keep going.* I was changing my truth, the thought that someone had planted into my head years ago. And I had to keep changing it every single day.

Sometimes your truth is a lie that you have let yourself believe. Maybe a family member, a friend, or a stranger said something bad to you that stuck with you for years. You don't have to believe it. It doesn't have to be *the* truth. Start today to look at those thoughts and tell yourself you are going to create a new truth about yourself. Don't allow yourself to talk negatively about yourself. Start believing, saying, and living the truth that you can be successful, healthy, and fit.

Mini-Challenge of the Day

Spend some time today reading the Bible. Write down five truths about yourself based on what the Scriptures tell us. Psalm 139 is a great place to start. Write down how wonderfully God made you and other statements from that passage so you can see the truth that God believes about you. Start by writing, "The truth is, I am..."

____

____

____

Tip of the Day

Never skip breakfast. You need energy to get you going, and eating at the start of your day will help you not to overeat later on.

Meal	Record Your Food & Water Intake for the Day	Calories
1		
2		
3		
4		
5		
	Total Calories	

Fitness Plan

Cardio activity: ____________________ Time: ________ Miles: ______

Intensity level (circle one): L M H

Strength training (circle): Lower body Upper body Core

My Thoughts

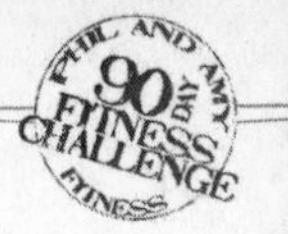

DAY 36—MINI GOALS

"A journey of a thousand miles
must begin with a single step."
Lao-tzu

A Note from Phil

Some time at the beginning of this "Challenge," you decided how much weight you wanted to lose. Maybe it was twenty, forty, or sixty pounds. I'm sure you've made considerable progress and have shed a couple (or more) pounds. Now is a good time to revisit your goal. First, you must figure out how many pounds you have yet to lose. Second, it's time to talk about how you're going to get there.

When you establish a long-term goal, there is one thing that will keep you on track to success—mini-goals. Mini-goals help you focus on your big goal and also help to make your big goal seem manageable. You don't want to set yourself up for failure or try to accomplish something that's not realistic.

During the "90-Day Fitness Challenge," Amy and I are committed to your process of gaining health. After all, we've been there ourselves. The way we've been able to lose all that weight and keep it off is by developing mini-goals along our journey. For example, drinking at least eight glasses of water a day is a realistic mini-goal that will improve your health. Eating lots of fresh fruit and vegetables is another mini-goal that can be measured and easily achieved. The same principle applies to exercise and rest. Whether your goal is to run a 5K race or compete in an Ironman Triathlon, list out mini-goals that will help you accomplish your ultimate goal.

When you look at the big picture of what you are trying to accomplish, it may seem like a daunting task. Creating mini-goals is the perfect antidote to that overwhelming pressure. I love the website www.coolrunning.com. On the site is a program called "Couch to 5K," which is designed for beginning runners to create a plan to get them off their couches and onto the road…running. Following this plan, step by step, takes a novice runner toward her dream of competing in races.

What about you? Consider your goals for your health, family, work, and any other area. It's time to design some mini-goals that will take you where you want to go!

Mini-Challenge of the Day

In the Mini-Challenge on Day 4, we asked you to look at your dream of getting fit and healthy and to create five mini-goals designed to help you get there. Go back and read what you wrote and examine your progress since then. Have you met or are you continuing to meet those goals? Are there any areas that could use some improvement or tweaking? Take some time and reevaluate those five things. In the spaces below, record whatever changes you need to make.

____

____

____

____

____

Tip of the Day

Sugar can hinder your weight loss and is found in so many things, so check the ingredient labels on the foods you are eating. If you see the words *high fructose corn syrup, corn syrup, sucrose, dextrose,* or *malto dextrose,* that is sugar so don't eat it.

Meal	Record Your Food & Water Intake for the Day	Calories
1		
2		
3		
4		
5		
	Total Calories	

Fitness Plan

Cardio activity: __________________ Time: _______ Miles: _____

Intensity level (circle one): L M H

Strength training (circle): Lower body Upper body Core

My Thoughts

___

___

___

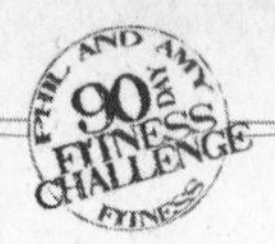

DAY 37—MAKE UP YOUR MIND

"A man who is master of himself can end a sorrow as easily as he can invent a pleasure. I don't want to be at the mercy of my emotions. I want to use them, to enjoy them, and to dominate them."

Oscar Wilde

A Word from Amy

My parents divorced when I was ten years old. I will never forget the wave of pain that washed over me when they delivered the bad news to my siblings and me. I specifically remember my mother saying that since I was the oldest, I had to be strong for my sisters and that she needed my help since my dad wasn't going to be with us anymore. In hindsight, I know that my mother was simply trying to make me feel important, but at the time I felt overwhelmed and overpowered by this huge burden of responsibility. It was as if I had to grow up at light speed. I couldn't afford to let my emotions get the best of me. I had to ignore my pain and stand strong. I believe this time in my life is when I made my first conscious decision to use food as my comforter.

After the divorce, my mother worked fifteen hours a day at the Dairy Queen restaurant that she owned. Many days, my sisters and I played all day in the back room or in the parking lot. I know she felt guilty for having to work as much as she did, so she would make it up to us by feeding us ice cream, burgers, and french fries.

As I got older, I got chubbier. And when someone would make fun of my weight, I would run to my old friend ice cream. Stress led to eating, eating led to more pounds, more pounds led to more stress, and...well, you get the idea. Being on national television and exposing myself in front of millions of people was stressful. Many times I felt like an acrobat falling off a tightrope without a safety net. Food had always been my safety net before, but it couldn't be that way anymore. I had to make up my mind not to turn to food when I was stressed. I had to make my mind more powerful than my emotions. It was a mental battle that took some time to win, but I did it. And so can you.

So how did I get there? First, I had to consciously recognize if I was going to the refrigerator, the grocery store, the bakery, or the snack basket because I was really hungry or because something was bothering me. Second, I learned when I was emotional to exchange eating for healthy things such as exercise, prayer, and having heart-to-hearts with Phil. Usually, I would convince myself that I wasn't really hungry and that I needed to go for a quick run or walk. Instead of grabbing the bagel, I put on my iPod and headed out the front door.

In this process, I was training myself to find a different way to handle my emotions. You need to do the same thing. Be aware of why you are eating. If you find yourself turning to food for comfort, recognize that you are doing this and substitute another activity. Only you can break the cycle.

Mini-Challenge of the Day

Just as an athlete needs to train her body and her mind to get into the best shape for a competition, we need to train our minds in the battle of the bulge. Think about your triggers for eating when you're not hungry. Now think of three activities you can do instead, such as going for a walk around the block, calling your best friend for support, getting on your knees and praying, and so on. Make it a point this week to recognize your triggers and use these substitutes instead.

Tip of the Day

When planning your meals for lunch and dinner, make sure your plate is half full of veggies.

Meal	Record Your Food & Water Intake for the Day	Calories
1		
2		
3		
4		
5		
	Total Calories	

Fitness Plan

Cardio activity: ____________________ Time: _______ Miles: _____

Intensity level (circle one): L M H

Strength training (circle): Lower body Upper body Core

My Thoughts

____

____

____

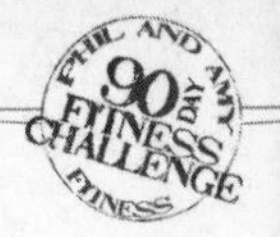

DAY 38—IT'S TIME TO CHANGE THE TAPE

"Ever tried? Ever failed? No matter.
Try again. Fail again. Fail better."
Samuel Beckett

A Word from Amy

Recently Phil and I were invited to the home of our mentors, who also happen to be close friends. These two are the kind of people I want to be like when I grow up, and I am thankful for their wisdom and example.

As we ate, the topic of cycling came up. Our hosts, who are in their fifties, are cyclists and regularly compete in triathlons. I admire the sport, but I have never seen myself as a cyclist. When I was eight years old, I literally ran over my sister with a bicycle and broke her leg. That memory popped up during the dinner conversation, and I realized I had always believed that if I got on a bike, I was going to hurt someone or myself. That memory became a replaying tape in my head. It was time to change that old tape that told me I couldn't be successful at biking and put in a new tape that told me I could.

Sometimes the tapes we play in our subconscious mind become the reality in our lives. If we believe we can never see ourselves as an athlete, then we will never be one. If we believe we can never get healthy, then we will never be healthy. If we believe we can't lose weight, we won't. If we believe we can't be successful, we won't.

Think about your own life. Take some time in prayer and let God show you some areas where you have allowed old tapes to dictate how you see yourself. It doesn't matter how long it's been since the tape's been rolling. It is never too late to change that tape. You can do more than you think. It's time to do great things, especially concerning your health. But remember what you gotta do first—change that tape!

Mini-Challenge of the Day

Think back to an instance in your life where someone you may have trusted or admired said something about you that hurt. Maybe you had a father who always called you "good for nothing." Maybe someone at work said you would always be fat. Whatever it is, write that statement down and below it, write down five positive statements about yourself (e.g., I am worth my health, I am beautiful, I am created in God's image and He doesn't make mistakes). Every time you are tempted to replay that negative statement, play these words of affirmation instead.

____

____

____

____

____

Tip of the Day

Don't eat too much red meat. Wherever you are, whether at home or at a restaurant, always choose the leanest cut of meat possible. Limit it to one or two servings a week.

Meal	Record Your Food & Water Intake for the Day	Calories
1		
2		
3		
4		
5		
	Total Calories	

Fitness Plan

Cardio activity: ____________________ Time: ________ Miles: ______

Intensity level (circle one): L M H

Strength training (circle): Lower body Upper body Core

My Thoughts

____

____

____

DAY 39—CHA-CHA-CHA-CHANGES

"Change is the only constant."
OLD PROVERB

A Word from Amy

Most of us like it when things are predictable. I love keeping a tight schedule and having order in my life. I am comfortable knowing what I'm doing and where I'm going. Don't get me wrong. I like a new adventure, but only if I plan it.

No one likes the kind of change that hits you out of left field—changes such as the loss of a job, an injury, or a friendship falling apart. In life, however, changes are inevitable, and how we react to them will determine whether we succeed or fail in our journey. In the past several years I have been through some severe changes. I have experienced a business failure, dealt with the autism diagnosis of our son, moved to a home that needed to be completely renovated, changed careers twice, and lost a hundred pounds.

I did not plan these changes. I had a completely different plan for my life. I always thought I would live in New York City and write for a magazine or become Mother of the Year, taking my kids to the park every day and caring for my family like June Cleaver. Neither of those things happened because God had another plan for my future. Did I want all those changes? Absolutely not! Have I learned through them? Most definitely.

Maybe you are faced with a change that you did not want. Maybe you lost a partner or have been laid off from your job. Maybe you can't communicate with a friend and the relationship is in jeopardy. Maybe you've had an accident and can't do some of the things you used to do. What are you going to do now?

I hope you will pick yourself up, learn from the experience, and adapt to your different life. Your outlook is the key, creating a mindset that's not afraid of change, but acknowledges it and adapts to it. If you look only at the negative of your current situation, you may never see the possibilities that the change may bring. When we lost our business, I was devastated. I look back now and understand that if it hadn't happened, we would have continued on a path that was not God's plan for us.

If we trust God and allow Him to lead us through our circumstances (no matter what they are or how difficult), we will ultimately fulfill our destined purpose. No matter what your journey may be, it's important to keep going.

Mini-Challenge of the Day

Set aside a few minutes today and surrender your plans and your life to God. Tell Him that you will trust Him, and ask Him to help you daily renew your mind and your thinking to encompass any changes that you are going through or that will come in the future.

Tip of the Day

I've said before that your legs are the largest muscle group in your body. When you do squats and lunges, you build those muscles, and muscles burn fat and calories. Squats and lunges don't require any gym equipment and are easy to do at home or even at the office.

Meal	Record Your Food & Water Intake for the Day	Calories
1		
2		
3		
4		
5		
	Total Calories	

Fitness Plan

Cardio activity: ______________________ Time: ________ Miles: ______

Intensity level (circle one): L M H

Strength training (circle): Lower body Upper body Core

My Thoughts

____

____

____

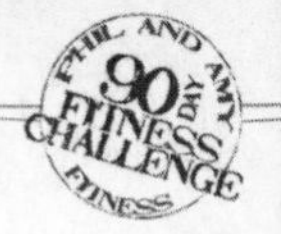

DAY 40—GIVING UP IS NOT AN OPTION

"Never, never, never give up."
WINSTON CHURCHILL

A Word from Amy

Those of you who watch *The Biggest Loser* may get the impression that the contestants' experience is so much easier than it actually is. Think about it. You see only two hours once a week of what took days to film. You can't feel what is going on through the television, so the producers try their best to show the highlights of the contestants struggles and triumphs.

If you think that the ranch is a magical fairyland of weight loss, you are very wrong. There are no hidden secrets that cause these people to lose dramatic amounts of weight. The results that you see on that show are because of large amounts of exercise and relearning how to eat only healthy foods. It's a process of detoxing the body from processed foods and sugars. It is physically, emotionally, and mentally demanding. And for most of us, it's the hardest thing we have ever done.

I say all of this, believe it or not, to encourage you. If you are having a difficult time in this journey, it's a sign that you're on the right track. If you are pushing yourself outside your comfort zone...good! If you have days where you struggle emotionally...great! This means you are in the middle of the battle instead of watching it from the sidelines.

Nothing worthwhile in life is without struggle. Just ask mothers if the road to childbirth is easy. One cannot imagine (unless you've been there) how painful it is to have a baby, but that same pain produces a miraculous life. Ask the players in the Super Bowl if the road to that game was an easy one. I'm sure they'll laugh in your face. Ask the presidential candidates if the road to the White House is easy. A year of nonstop travel, speeches, and fund-raising? What do you think?

If you're finding the road to health difficult, then that just proves great things are on the horizon. Never give up because something is hard. Keep going until you reach your goal, because that is your reward. Many people give up right when their breakthrough is about to come. If you think you've hit a plateau in your weight, keep eating right. If you can't see any results in your fitness work, don't quit. If you don't think you can get through the next few days, tell yourself otherwise. Don't give up on your dream. You've come too far!

Mini-Challenge of the Day

If you feel yourself on the verge of giving up this "Challenge," make a phone call to someone who is fully supportive of your adventure. Tell this person you need some encouragement. Don't be afraid of being vulnerable or embarrassed. We all need a cheerleader when we face tough challenges.

Tip of the Day

Hummus is one of our favorite dips with vegetables. Hummus is made out of chickpeas, tahini, and lemon juice. It's affordable and delicious with carrot sticks, celery sticks, or red pepper slices.

Meal	Record Your Food & Water Intake for the Day	Calories
1		
2		
3		
4		
5		
	Total Calories	

Fitness Plan

Cardio activity: ____________________ Time: ________ Miles: ______

Intensity level (circle one): L M H

Strength training (circle): Lower body Upper body Core

My Thoughts

____

____

____

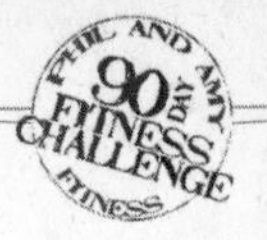

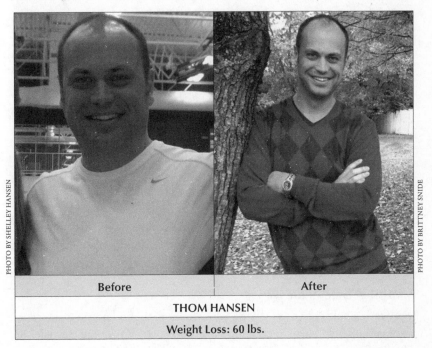

DAY 41—**TAKE CARE OF YOUR HEALTH**

"A man too busy to take care of his health is like a mechanic too busy to take care of his tools."
SPANISH PROVERB

It has been a delight to witness the progress of Thom's journey. He lost so much weight and became a whole new person, inside and out. Read what he has to say.

PHOTO BY SHELLEY HANSEN

PHOTO BY BRITTNEY SNIDE

Before	After
THOM HANSEN	
Weight Loss: 60 lbs.	

"I was a fit kid through elementary school and into my junior high years. I always scored high on the fitness tests, and in seventh grade, my physical education teacher asked me to join the track team. At my very first track meet, I injured myself, and that's when my weight struggle began.

"I was bedridden for a while and began to pack on the pounds. I went through high school not exercising and eating all the wrong things. I ballooned up to 280 pounds. I lived for so long at that weight, I became used to my size and didn't want to do anything about it.

"I got married in 2000 and divorced two years later. I coped by becoming an emotional eater. My routine was the same most nights. I drank two liters of Coke before bedtime and took a trip to Dunkin' Donuts at midnight to eat four donuts with some milk. It wasn't unusual for me to polish off an entire pizza in one sitting. I knew I wasn't living a healthy lifestyle, but I kept on living that way.

"In January 2008 I saw a post on Facebook about a fitness challenge that was going to be held at a new gym in town. I called up some friends to go with me. We were the first ones to arrive at the gym and very excited to hear what Phil and Amy were going to tell us. We were hoping to walk away with a whole lot of information that could make us healthier.

"I listened to every word Phil and Amy had to say and even had my measurements taken (how embarrassing!). I was scared to share my stats with my friends, but I had to because now they were my accountability partners. The 'Challenge' was an incredible experience, and I saw results fast. I lost eight pounds the first week. All I did was eat healthier, drink tons of water, and start exercising. As each week passed, I lost more weight. During the 'Challenge,' I lost thirty-nine pounds.

"I set some different goals for myself and kept on with the 'Challenge' after the ninety days was over. I have now lost a total of sixty pounds, and have run six 5K races and one 8K. When I stepped on the treadmill when I started this program, I could barely run a quarter of a mile. Today, I work out almost every day, sleep seven to eight hours a night, and eat the right foods. I am loving life with this new body that I have. I'm gaining muscles in new places and people always comment on how I look like a different person."

Mini-Challenge of the Day

Watch an old episode of *The Biggest Loser.* You can find previous shows on the Internet. It will help to encourage and inspire you. Learn one new idea or exercise from that show and apply it to you today.

Tip of the Day

Drinking water regularly will keep the brain working properly. Studies have shown that not drinking enough water can cause headaches, migraines, chronic fatigue syndrome, and depression. So make sure you drink enough water.

Meal	Record Your Food & Water Intake for the Day	Calories
1		
2		
3		
4		
5		
	Total Calories	

Fitness Plan

Cardio activity: ____________________ Time: ________ Miles: ______

Intensity level (circle one): L M H

Strength training (circle): Lower body Upper body Core

My Thoughts

____

____

____

The Importance of Planning and Organizing: Strategizing for Success

Never underestimate the power of planning and organizing to keep you on the right path to better health. In this section you'll learn tips for making food for the whole week, creating to-do lists, and organizing your kitchen. This is the week you'll get rid of all your junk food (yes, you can do it, if you haven't done it already), so get those trash bags ready. You'll even learn how to be prepared when you're traveling and how to organize your new lifestyle to keep your children involved too.

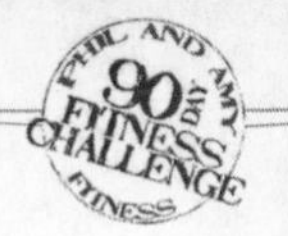

DAY 42—IT TAKES WORK

"There are no secrets to success.
It is the result of preparation, hard work,
and learning from failure."
Colin Powell

A Note from Phil

I'm not going to lie to you. Making your health a priority takes planning and focus. We've already told you that it's of the utmost importance that you eat every three to four hours. As you start training, your metabolism picks up, and you will know when it is time to eat again because you will be hungry three hours after your last meal. Did you know that many people who struggle with weight don't often feel hungry? This is a telltale sign that their metabolism is not working properly.

It can be challenging to find healthy and tasty food when you're on the go. This is why you need to prepare meals and snacks ahead of time and take them with you wherever you go. This will prevent you from being caught without food when hunger strikes. Amy and I take one day of the week, usually on Saturday or Sunday, and cook at least five days' worth of food for lunches, dinners, and snacks. (We don't premake breakfast since toast, eggs, cereal, or oatmeal take only a few minutes to prepare in the morning.)

We buy big bags of chicken, brown rice, whole wheat pasta, and various vegetables at a wholesale club. These are the staples that most of our menus revolve around. We prepare the chicken in different light marinades or spices and then either grill, bake, or broil them. We cook the rice and pasta in larger pots and set those aside. We quickly steam a bunch of vegetables such as squash, broccoli, carrots, zucchini, mushrooms, onions, and peppers. Using those staples, we make a few different combinations, and then divide them into storage containers for quick use throughout the week. We have even put labels on each container with the calorie count for that meal so we take the guesswork out of calorie counting.

Snacks are easy. We put almonds, Wasa crackers, fruit, and other snack items in individual baggies so they are easy to grab as we are running out the door.

While preparing this food takes about three to four hours on the weekend, it's an important step to eating success. During the busy workweek, you will always have food ready to eat three to four times a day. There will be no need for excuses to stop at McDonald's. You'll also save money buying food in bulk. By spending some time preparing, your body will be thinner and your wallet fatter.

Mini-Challenge of the Day

Pick a day this week and cook your meals for the next five days. Prepare a meal plan using our suggestions or meals from a healthy cookbook. Ask a friend to help.

Tip of the Day

Feel like overeating? An acronym to remember is HALT. Being too Hungry, Angry, Lonely, or Tired are conditions that leave us more vulnerable to the temptations to binge. Instead of eating impulsively, do a check—Do you need some rest? Do you need to call a friend? Did something tick you off today? Did you skip a meal? These four conditions are strong triggers that will tempt us to overeat, so pay attention to yourself.

Meal	Record Your Food & Water Intake for the Day	Calories
1		
2		
3		
4		
5		
	Total Calories	

Fitness Plan

Cardio activity: ______________________ Time: ________ Miles: ______

Intensity level (circle one): L M H

Strength training (circle): Lower body Upper body Core

My Thoughts

____

____

____

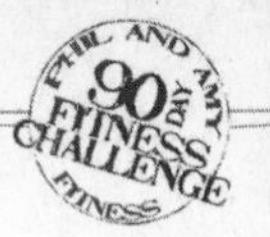

DAY 43—TIME MANAGEMENT

"Time is what we want most, but what we use worst."
William Penn

A Word from Amy

How many times have you said to yourself "I don't have time to exercise" or "I don't have time to cook all my meals" or "I just don't have time…period." I hear these statements all the time. I even used to say these things myself. But everyone has the same twenty-four hours in a day. I have twenty-four hours in a day. You have twenty-four hours in a day. The president of the United States has twenty-four hours in a day. No one has more time than anyone else. The amount of time we have isn't the issue; it's how we use our time.

We spend so much time on things that aren't producing any positive results in our lives. I used to spend hours every night watching television. My life revolved around the nightly TV schedule and what I was going to eat while watching. I wasted hours of my life that could have been spent more productively. I could have been exercising during that time or getting the right amount of sleep or reading books on health.

Think about your own life. How are you spending the twenty-fours each day that God has given you? I read that the average American watches four hours of TV a day. Four hours is a lot of time that could be used to do things that are life-giving or life-changing, not just sitting in front of a screen being entertained. Maybe you spend your time doing other things that aren't productive, such as surfing the web, shopping, reading tabloid magazines, or chatting on the phone. Be honest with yourself about how much time you spend doing things that only waste time.

Have you ever had a friend call you up at the last minute and invite you to come to their vacation home for the weekend? Isn't it amazing how quickly we can rearrange our schedules, get the dog taken care of, pack a suitcase for every member of the family, straighten up the house, gas up the car, and hit the road because it's an invitation to do something fun?

Well, guess what? I have a ticket to a new life waiting for you. You just have to rearrange your schedule a little and make a few changes. How badly do you want to make the change? How badly do you want to be in better shape? How badly do you want to be in better health? Make time by eliminating the things you know you don't need to be doing. Use your day wisely.

Mini-Challenge of the Day

Keep track of your time today. From the minute you wake up to the time you go to bed, write down everything you do and how long it takes. At the end of the day, review what you have written down and see where you can make some changes. Notice where you are wasting time and make a commitment to stop doing these things.

Tip of the Day

Take containers of flavored yogurt and put them in the freezer. Frozen yogurt is a delicious and healthy substitute for ice cream.

Meal	Record Your Food & Water Intake for the Day	Calories
1		
2		
3		
4		
5		
	Total Calories	

Fitness Plan

Cardio activity: ______________________ Time: ________ Miles: ______

Intensity level (circle one): L M H

Strength training (circle): Lower body Upper body Core

My Thoughts

____

____

____

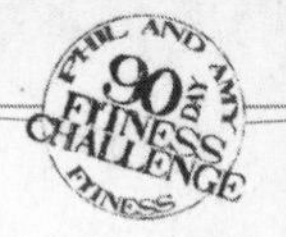

DAY 44—MAKING LISTS

"The key is not to prioritize what's on your schedule, but to schedule your priorities."
Stephen Covey

A Note from Phil

Everyone who knows me can tell you I probably have some form of ADD, although I've never been officially diagnosed. Though I consider myself a task-oriented person, I am also unstructured (think organized chaos) and love change (sometimes too much). It was always tough for me to have structure in my health habits, but on the ranch I had no choice. The lifestyle there provided us with structure for most of our day in our eating and exercise routines. This was new to me, but I adapted.

When I came home, all of that structure was gone. I learned very quickly that I had to take what I learned and integrate a routine into my daily life. The key to my success was organization and prioritization. I knew every class at every gym I worked out in. I knew every calorie that went into my mouth.

Maybe it seems a little obsessive-compulsive, but keeping lists will help you keep track of your priorities and meet your goals.

If you write your daily tasks on paper, you are more likely to get them done and less likely to waste time. I keep a long to-do list that I add to as needed. I prioritize the list by asking myself, "Does this move me closer to my goal or will it distract me?" "Is this something I need to do or just something I would like to do?" I find that if I am accountable to the list, then my life is more orderly and I get more things done.

You will find that you need to schedule time for workouts, eating more regularly, as well as all the other things you have to do in a day. Start by making lists for the different goals you've set for yourself. Then, every morning, look at those lists and pick the top ten things you need to get done in order of importance. Ask yourself the same questions I ask myself so you can determine what you need to do today and what can wait for another day.

Get organized and meet your goals. What are you waiting for?

Mini-Challenge of the Day

Every evening before you go to bed, write in a notebook at least five things that you absolutely must get done the next day. Look at the list when you wake up, and you'll be ready to carry out your tasks for the day.

Tip of the Day

Here's a trick to help you cut calories. Eat the low-calorie items on your plate first, then graduate to the next item. For example, start out by eating the salads, veggies, and broth soups; eat meats and starches last. By the time you get to the last two, you won't be that hungry.

Meal	Record Your Food & Water Intake for the Day	Calories
1		
2		
3		
4		
5		
	Total Calories	

Fitness Plan

Cardio activity: ____________________ Time: ________ Miles: ______

Intensity level (circle one): L M H

Strength training (circle): Lower body Upper body Core

My Thoughts

____

____

____

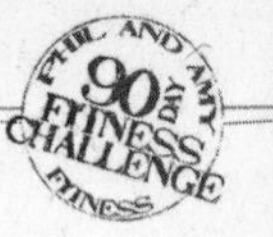

DAY 45—WHAT ABOUT THE CHILDREN?

"Train up a child in the way he should go,
even when he is old he will not depart from it."
Proverbs 22:6 NASB

A Word from Amy

Many parents who begin a weight-loss plan worry that if they take time to exercise and eat well, it will take time away from their kids. I also discovered that many mothers feel guilty when they eliminate the sweets and snacks their kids enjoy. How do you plan your healthy lifestyle and make those changes for your children too?

When we came home from the ranch, we were still in competition for four more months until the weigh-in at the season finale. Phil and I decided to immediately remove all the junk food from our house. We did not give our kids a choice. Did they whine and complain? Of course! But they quickly learned to adapt. We discovered that the little guys were always hungry because their sugar-loaded diets never gave them the nutrients they needed. Now they know healthy delicious meals give them more energy and they feel great. They also appreciate the times when they are allowed to have desserts. Once in a while we will go out for frozen yogurt, and it's such a treat for them.

We never forced our boys to exercise or they would learn that exercise was a chore. Instead, we decided to just be an example for them and hoped they would follow in our footsteps. I noticed that when Phil and I came back from the gym, we always had more energy, and our kids would respond to us in a more positive way. We started to ask them if they wanted to join us in activities. First, we took walks around the block after dinner. Then we encouraged them to run a 5K with us for charity. We invited them to the gym to work out, especially if there was a kid's event going on there. Gradually, we noticed them being more active. Our oldest son joined the cross-country team at his school and our middle son dropped ten pounds. We learned when it comes to exercise, your children will learn more by what you do than what you say. Your plan for better health will influence their own.

Always remember that you are the parent, and they will follow as you lead. Lead them down the healthy path.

Mini-Challenge of the Day

Today, make a list of three activities you think your kids would enjoy doing with you. Choose one activity for them to do with you today. Ask them about the other two next week.

Tip of the Day

Eat before you go grocery shopping. The worst thing you can do is go to the supermarket hungry. You never want to go to the store when you've skipped a meal or when you want to pick up a few random things before coming home for dinner. This can lead to impulse buying. Go grocery shopping when you are full.

Meal	Record Your Food & Water Intake for the Day	Calories
1		
2		
3		
4		
5		
	Total Calories	

Fitness Plan

Cardio activity: ____________________ Time: ________ Miles: ______

Intensity level (circle one): L M H

Strength training (circle): Lower body Upper body Core

My Thoughts

____

____

____

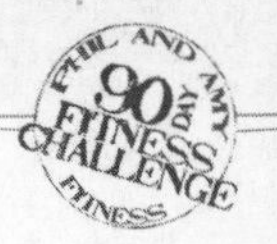

DAY 46—IDEAS FOR TRAVELING

"Planning is bringing the future into the present so that you can do something about it now."

ALAN LAKEIN

A Note from Phil

Amy and I travel often for speaking engagements. While it's more difficult to maintain your healthy diet when you travel, it's definitely still possible. You don't have to blow it when you're away just because you're not in the safe comfort of your own home. You just need to be prepared before you leave on your trip. We plan our food and workouts before we leave the house. Here are some suggestions for you based on the traveling habits we've acquired.

To start, try to book a hotel with a gym. If that's not possible, call ahead to see if the hotel is close to quiet roads for walking. The closer everything is to the hotel, the easier it will be for you to stick to your routine. You don't want to spend thirty minutes driving to a nearby gym or hiking trail because, chances are, you'll find an excuse not to go.

Remember, you can always work out in your hotel room. I always pack resistance bands and a jump rope in my luggage. Or put some music on and dance around for thirty minutes—that will burn as many calories as a brisk walk. Here are some other ideas for exercising in your hotel room:

- jumping jacks
- lunges
- push-ups
- sit-ups and crunches
- triceps dips

As far as your diet, accept that you will probably be eating out a lot. Apply the same guidelines for eating out that we've given you in the "Eat to Live" chapter. Before you leave, pack a few baggies of snacks to help keep you eating as healthy as possible. Bring some nuts, protein bars, or apples. If it's a quick trip, bring some yogurt, celery and peanut butter, or mixed fruit. Here are more tips:

- Instead of bread, use lettuce. Even if you have to eat at a fast-food chain, ask for a grilled chicken or roast beef sandwich with lettuce on the side. Then eat your protein wrapped in lettuce, tomatoes, and onions without the bread.

- Order a grilled chicken salad. Watch out for creamy dressings, though. Always ask for oil and vinegar or use light dressings. Salads can be found in almost any airport.
- Traveling can be stressful. Don't use the stress as an excuse to treat yourself with unhealthy foods. Use travel as an opportunity to stick to your healthy plan by making good choices and staying flexible.

Mini-Challenge of the Day

Look at your calendar and find the next time you will travel. What are three things you can do to prepare now to keep your diet on track? For example, how many baggies of snacks do you think you will need to prepare and take with you?

Tip of the Day

Eating healthy doesn't mean a bigger budget. Clip coupons every weekend. Buy the poultry, fish, or meats that are on sale this week. Look for the "Buy 2 Get 1 Free" specials. Don't worry about the brands that much, focus on the ingredients instead. Usually the generic or supermarket brand is just as good as the popular brand.

Meal	Record Your Food & Water Intake for the Day	Calories
1		
2		
3		
4		
5		
	Total Calories	

Fitness Plan

Cardio activity: ______________________ Time: ________ Miles: ______

Intensity level (circle one): L M H

Strength training (circle): Lower body Upper body Core

My Thoughts

____

____

____

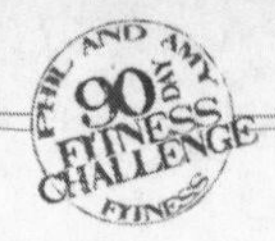

DAY 47—GET RID OF THE JUNK

"Out of sight, out of mind."

A Note from Phil

It's time to clean out your pantry and refrigerator. If you did this already, congratulations! But maybe since that initial purge things have accumulated in your house that you need to get rid of. If you didn't clean out your pantry and fridge yet, it's time to do it. Don't allow the following excuses to keep you from having a healthy home:

- I don't eat this stuff, but I have to keep it for the kids.
- I will just keep a few things for the high-calorie day.
- The food costs so much money, I feel guilty just throwing it away.
- I can't survive without a little ________________ (chocolate, chips, candy).
- I have to keep some of these foods here for when I have company.

These excuses are one of the many roadblocks that keep you from your dreams. Remove the food and you remove this roadblock.

Let's get started. First, throw out all the junk food. This includes cookies, chips, candy, ice cream, crackers, sodas, sugary cereals, and cakes. Then get rid of the meal-in-a-box packages and white starches. I'm talking about pasta meals, boxed potato meals, macaroni and cheese, white potatoes, white bread, white pasta, and white rice. Your panty and fridge must be getting close to empty by now. But we're not done just yet. Take a look at the labels on the foods that are left. Throw out anything high in sodium. These are usually canned soups, canned pasta meals, and canned vegetables. Finally, get rid of regular table salt and high-sodium seasonings and dressings such as soy sauce and ranch salad dressing. Do you still have any unnatural sweeteners or foods with sugar in them? Throw them out.

Don't be alarmed if your kitchen is empty. The less junk you have, the more dramatic the change will be in your health.

Now you're ready to do some shopping. It's time to go out and buy foods that will give you the body you've always dreamed about and the energy level you wish you had. Refer to appendix B for foods you should buy.

In case you're the only one in your family embarking on this "Challenge," you might not have the support you need. You can compromise until the rest of your family gets more comfortable with the changes. Keep some junk in a locked cupboard. Choose the highest shelf in the kitchen. This way it's still available for your family but not easily accessible to you. But give yourself a deadline, perhaps two months, when you will throw even that food out.

Mini-Challenge of the Day

No more excuses. This is your day to clean out your pantry and fridge. Get that big trash bin and get rid of that junk.

Tip of the Day

Include at least one legume meal per week, such as tofu or baked beans. Legumes are a great meat alternative and are very filling. Look online for some tasty legume recipes.

Meal	Record Your Food & Water Intake for the Day	Calories
1		
2		
3		
4		
5		
	Total Calories	

Fitness Plan

Cardio activity: ____________________ Time: ________ Miles: ______

Intensity level (circle one): L M H

Strength training (circle): Lower body Upper body Core

My Thoughts

____

____

____

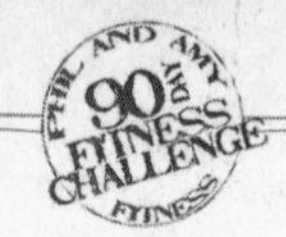

DAY 48—ORGANIZING YOUR FOOD

"The ability to simplify means to eliminate the unnecessary so that the necessary may speak."
HANS HOFFMAN

A Word from Amy

When it comes to food, it pays to be organized. Before you go food shopping, make a list. This will help you remember what you need and stick to your budget. Don't leave home without it. Next, organize your shopping list into categories. Group all the vegetables together, all the meats, and all the dairy. You don't want to waste time going back and forth through the entire store plus you'll only get tempted by the thousands of choices you pass by. If possible, shop as much as you can in the perimeter of the store. The aisles have most of the processed foods.

When you get home, don't unload your groceries just wherever you find room. We have our pantry and fridge organized in such a way that when we look inside, we know in less than a minute what we can put together for a meal. If you're like me and don't have enough time in the day, this is critical. Here are some ideas:

- Group similar foods together. Put the cereals and oatmeal on one shelf. Store the nuts and healthy snacks on another shelf. Put the rice, pasta, and bread on another. Put all the salad dressings in the fridge door.
- If you can't see it, you don't know what you have. We used to overstock our shelves so much that during spring cleaning, we'd find tons of food in the very back that had already passed its expiration date. Leave some room on your shelves so you can see what you have.
- Do you have too many foods to store that are the same? Keep them in separate places. For example, if you bought two large bags of rice, put one in the pantry and put the overstock in another room (the basement or laundry room) so you don't clutter your shelves.
- If you can, label your shelves. Your family might think you've gone overboard, but that's okay. Also, if your whole family knows where everything goes, then they can help you unpack the groceries.

- Put the smaller items in the front, unless they are used every day. In the fridge, we try to shelve the smaller items in the front so we can see to the back of the fridge. However, when it's a gallon of milk or a carton of orange juice, we keep those in the front since we use them every day.

Mini-Challenge of the Day

Attach a shopping list pad on the fridge with a magnet. Keep a pen nearby. Write down whatever you need to buy as soon as you know you need it.

Tip of the Day

Instead of whole milk, switch to 1 percent or skim. If you drink one eight-ounce glass a day, you'll lose five pounds in a year by making this simple change.

Meal	Record Your Food & Water Intake for the Day	Calories
1		
2		
3		
4		
5		
	Total Calories	

Fitness Plan

Cardio activity: ____________________ Time: ________ Miles: ______

Intensity level (circle one): L M H

Strength training (circle): Lower body Upper body Core

My Thoughts

____

____

____

DAY 49—NOT ACCORDING TO PLAN

"If you have made mistakes, there is always another chance for you. You may have a fresh start any moment you choose, for this thing we call 'failure' is not the falling down, but the staying down."

MARY PICKFORD, ACTRESS

A Word from Amy

We've talked a lot about planning and organizing. Planning and organizing your day. Planning and organizing your workouts. Planning and organizing what you're going to eat. But what happens when our plans don't go according to our plans? Life happens. Sometimes our kids get sick. Or we have a major deadline at work. Or we have a traumatic event that flips our world upside down. When these things happen, even though we are committed to keeping our plans on this "Challenge," sometimes we simply can't.

Don't beat yourself up. Getting off course because of major interruptions (or even just getting off course because you've slipped up) doesn't mean you've failed. It usually means that you need to make a small shift somewhere. All my life I struggled with an "all or nothing" mentality. If I couldn't do something all the way, then I would quit.

You have to avoid this destructive attitude when you're trying to live a healthy lifestyle. We will inevitably have a tough day from time to time. It's gonna happen. And when it does, we need to talk to ourselves. I know it's been said that talking to yourself is a sign of insanity, but I have found it to be an effective way to change my mindset.

When those tough days come and your plans fall to the wayside, just tell yourself that you're going to give yourself a few days to get through ________ (whatever crisis you are going through), and then it will be time to get back on track. Give yourself a mental vacation so you don't quit altogether.

No one is perfect or has a perfect life, so why should you be an exception? People of true character get back up when they fall down. So get up, dust yourself off, and get back in the game.

Mini-Challenge of the Day

If you are going through something today that has been a catalyst for getting off course, spend some time in prayer and meditation. Ask God to get you through. Forgive yourself and remind yourself that you will get back on the wagon and ride the "Challenge" out. If you have not had one of these moments yet, be prepared. If and when you do, remember these words: forgive yourself, give yourself a pep talk, and keep moving forward.

Tip of the Day

Have you tried taking a yoga class? Yoga is an easy way to relax, reduce stress, and boost your health. It helps add flexibility to your joints and muscles and helps clear your mind. Check out classes at your local gym or community center.

Meal	Record Your Food & Water Intake for the Day	Calories
1		
2		
3		
4		
5		
	Total Calories	

Fitness Plan

Cardio activity: ______________________ Time: ________ Miles: ______

Intensity level (circle one): L M H

Strength training (circle): Lower body Upper body Core

My Thoughts

____

____

____

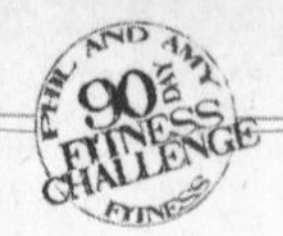

DAY 50—LOSING WEIGHT SAVES LIVES

"It's not hard to make decisions
when you know what your values are."
Roy Disney

This sweet young woman touched our heart when we heard her story. This is just another example of how focusing on bettering your health will not only change but can even save your life. Read the beautiful email she sent us.

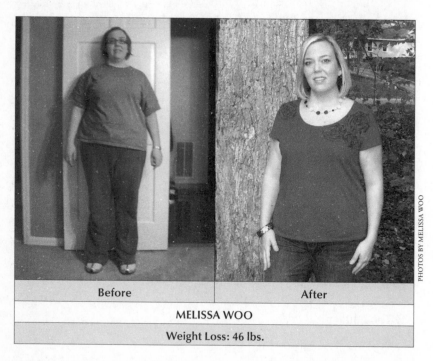

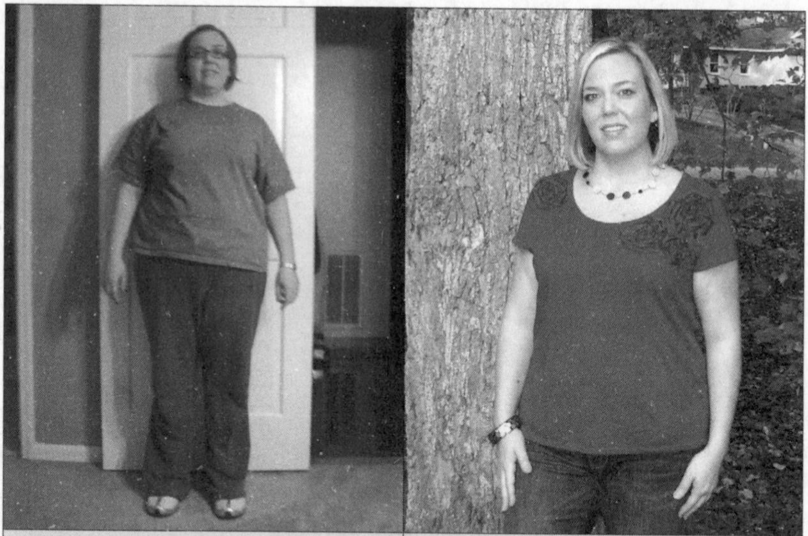

Before	After
MELISSA WOO	
Weight Loss: 46 lbs.	

PHOTOS BY MELISSA WOO

"I have been a fan of *The Biggest Loser* since Season 1. When I found out that Phil and Amy Parham were hosting a '90-Day Fitness Challenge' near where I live, I was quick to sign up and so excited to meet them in person.

"Like many people, I have tried several plans to lose weight, only to be disappointed and fail. As I listened to Amy and Phil's story, I began to believe in myself and decided this was the program for me. There was something different about this challenge than any other program I had tried. I thought if they could give me a guide to follow and help me along the way, it would help me mentally, physically, and spiritually.

"I started working out, which was so new to me. After three months I had lost ten pounds. I wanted to jump start my program, so I called the Parhams' at-home trainer D.J. Jordan. I quickly learned that D.J. 'don't play.' He is very patient, but he demands results.

"So far I have lost forty-six pounds, and I hope to lose a total of seventy-five pounds. For the first time I feel as though I am in control of my life. Since starting the 'Challenge' I have learned to eat smaller portions and to enjoy healthier choices. This is now a lifestyle for me and my wonderful family, who I love more than anything in this world. Amy and Phil have helped me realize that I am a winner not a quitter."

Mini-Challenge of the Day

Think about ways taking care of your health can save your life. Maybe you have high blood pressure and making better choices in your diet will lower your numbers. Maybe you have a heart condition that can be alleviated through exercise. Whatever the case may be, focus today on your health and the rewards of making good decisions.

Tip of the Day

Not only does regular exercise help you feel and look better, it can also reduce your risk of catching a cold. Just another incentive to get moving.

Meal	Record Your Food & Water Intake for the Day	Calories
1		
2		
3		
4		
5		
	Total Calories	

Fitness Plan

Cardio activity: ______________________ Time: ________ Miles: ______

Intensity level (circle one): L M H

Strength training (circle): Lower body Upper body Core

My Thoughts

____

____

____

Empowerment: Realizing Your Own Strength

You are much stronger than you know. This week, we'll take the time to reflect on your inner processes, your strengths, and your hidden challenges. We'll help you discover the true treasure you are and help to set you free to become what God knows you can be.

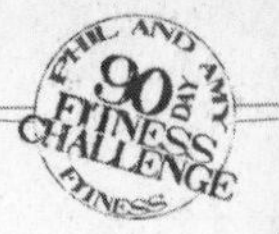

DAY 51—GOING THROUGH THE PROCESS

"Your life is the sum result of all the choices you make, both consciously and unconsciously. If you can control the process of choosing, you can take control of all aspects of your life. You can find the freedom that comes from being in charge of yourself."

Robert F. Bennett

A Word from Amy

Every time I ask Rhett, our autistic son, to do something, he has a process that he has to go through to be able to do what I ask. For example, if we tell him to do his homework, he yells at the top of his lungs, "I don't want to do my homework!" After he yells, he calmly walks over to his book bag and gets out his homework to work on it. He does the same thing when I tell him to take a bath, take out the trash, or any other request we make of him. It's almost as if he has to loudly announce his opposition before he agrees to do what we asked him to do.

Many of us do the same thing when we are told we need to do something. Our doctor says we need to lose weight, and we find ourselves at the Burger King drive-thru immediately after the appointment. We know we need to exercise, but instead we lie on the sofa. We might even get to the parking lot of the gym, but we leave before we actually get through the front door. We all know what we need to do to be healthy, but we dig in our heels as long as we can before we finally admit we have no choice but to get healthy.

Right now you are fifty-one days into the "Challenge." Maybe you've hit a plateau. Maybe you're bored with your workouts. Maybe you're sick of eating healthy food. Don't give up. Be empowered and stop fighting the urge that tells you to quit. Here are some tips to embrace the "Challenge" and continue on your way.

- Accept the fact that the road to health is seldom an easy one. The things in life that are the most valuable require the most sacrifice. Just because things get hard doesn't mean that's a sign to quit. These are the times to prove just how strong you are.
- Tell yourself that eating healthy and exercising is your idea. Convince yourself it's your choice, not something someone else is telling you to do.

- Remind yourself that this is a process and not an event. Take one day at a time and celebrate every small success because they will eventually add up to big victories.
- List the things that will be different in your life when you get healthy. Smaller sizes in clothes, more energy, playing sports you've never played before, feeling confident—these are all good ones to write down.

Empower yourself with these tips and keep going. Ninety days will be here before you know it.

Mini-Challenge of the Day

What are two things that you know you should be doing that you've been tempted not to do? Write them down. Why do you think you are rebelling against the things that will bring you closer to your goal? Take time to think about your process for achieving health and fitness and embrace it fully.

____

____

____

Tip of the Day

If you don't feel like exercising one day, use the twenty minute rule. Just tell yourself you'll work out for twenty minutes. It's a short time frame but long enough to see benefits. Chances are, you'll end up having a forty-five minute session because you feel so good. Use this tool to negotiate your way to the gym and at least start your workout.

Meal	Record Your Food & Water Intake for the Day	Calories
1		
2		
3		
4		
5		
	Total Calories	

Fitness Plan

Cardio activity: ______________________ Time: ________ Miles: ______

Intensity level (circle one): L M H

Strength training (circle): Lower body Upper body Core

My Thoughts

____

____

____

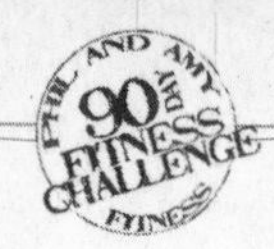

DAY 52—LIFE IS GOOD

"The more you praise and celebrate your life,
the more there is in life to celebrate."
OPRAH WINFREY

A Word from Amy

Have you ever seen someone wearing those "Life is Good" T-shirts when life wasn't going good for you that day? I bet you wanted to smack the person wearing it, right? We all have bad days. That's why it's so important to focus on our blessings. Our minds are like a magnifying glass. What we focus on gets bigger. Make it a habit to remind yourself of the victories and blessings in your life. They don't even have to be related to weight loss.

When I'm feeling down, I start thinking about all the things I have done right. First, I think about my kids, who are wonderful, funny, loving, and giving. In spite of having us as parents (I'm sure all parents feel that way every now and again), my kids are turning out pretty darn good. I then think of other blessings in my life. I was blessed to have wonderful parents. I think about everything I've experienced being on the show. So many millions of people wish they could have had my experience, and I was blessed to have been one of the ones chosen. If it's a really bad day, I continue to think like this until I am out of my funk. Trust me, it works.

You might have had some sort of setback. Maybe you got sick and couldn't work out for a while or you goofed one day with your eating. While you are powerless to change your circumstances, you can empower yourself and change your attitude. Count your blessings. Be grateful for how far you've come. Appreciate your hard work.

Accept that there are things in life you can and can't control. Sometimes things just won't go your way. Count your blessings and go with the flow. And if you're able to take control and change things to make your life better and happier, then do it. Get back on track with healthy eating if you slipped up. Get back into the gym if you haven't gone in a while. But most of all, remember all the blessings God has given you—your friends, your family, the opportunity to be part of this "Challenge," and the very life you are living.

Mini-Challenge of the Day

Count your blessings. Like the old gospel song says, "Name them one by one." List at least five victories or blessings in your life. Today, focus on those and eliminate all thoughts of failure.

____

____

____

Tip of the Day

Don't compare yourself with others. The only person you should be competing with is yourself. I still struggle with this from time to time because I work out with athletes and people half my age. I could compare myself to them, but instead, I focus on my personal goals. As long as I improve my workouts and push myself daily, I am happy.

Meal	Record Your Food & Water Intake for the Day	Calories
1		
2		
3		
4		
5		
	Total Calories	

Fitness Plan

Cardio activity: ________________ Time: ______ Miles: _____

Intensity level (circle one): L M H

Strength training (circle): Lower body Upper body Core

My Thoughts

____

____

____

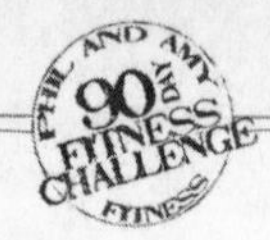

DAY 53—PRISON BREAK

"I count him braver who overcomes his desires than him who conquers his enemies; for the hardest victory is over self."
Aristotle

A Word from Amy

Recently I was walking through my house, and suddenly I remembered what it felt like to be a prisoner in my own body. Because I've been on my journey to get healthy for almost two years now, it's easy to forget the desperation I used to feel. All the emotions of feeling trapped, winded, worn down, and sick have settled into the dust.

I used to be so tired when my children asked me to do something. Getting up the motivation to go anywhere (even the mall) was a challenge. I would avoid going up the stairs because I would be out of breath when I made it up there. While the way things used to be is a distant memory now, I never want to forget how far I've come. One of the biggest motivators and joys for me is to remember what it felt like to be a prisoner in my body and what it feels like to have the chains of poor health, excess weight, and unhealthy habits broken.

You are in the process of making a prison break. You've already come so far, and I am so proud of you. Keep up the good work and keep on going. Remember, every day that you choose to exercise and eat healthy, you are chipping away, bit by bit, at the chains of poor health. Every time you choose water instead of soda, choose to take the stairs instead of the elevator, or choose to pay attention to your body instead of ignoring signs of exhaustion, you are one step closer to true freedom.

As you continue the "90-Day Fitness Challenge," don't beat yourself up for your shortcomings. What are you going to do about them? That's what matters.

God has a plan for your life that is far above what you have for it. While you are trying to figure out how to achieve your dream of better health, He is thinking about how you can fulfill the great purpose He has for you. Dream bigger, reach higher, and break free of your chains. Let these words give you the strength to follow through and reach your goals.

Mini-Challenge of the Day

Think of how an unhealthy body is your prison. What are three ways your body limits you because you are overweight or not in shape? Use this as a motivation to reach your goals. Your body should be the tool you use to do what God has called you to do. It should not be your prison.

____

____

____

Tip of the Day

If you exercise after work, bring your gym bag with you and go straight from your job to the gym. Don't convince yourself to stop at home first and then work out. Chances are, you'll come home and find fifty things to do that will distract you from getting to the gym.

Meal	Record Your Food & Water Intake for the Day	Calories
1		
2		
3		
4		
5		
	Total Calories	

Fitness Plan

Cardio activity: ____________________ Time: ________ Miles: ______

Intensity level (circle one): L M H

Strength training (circle): Lower body Upper body Core

My Thoughts

____

____

____

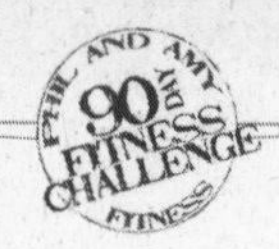

DAY 54—NO MORE PITY PARTIES

"Feeling sorry for yourself, and your present condition, is not only a waste of energy but the worst habit you could possibly have."

DALE CARNEGIE

A Word from Amy

I remember how tired I felt when I was losing weight. Not only was I physically tired, but I was tired of working out, tired of eating right, tired of following my plan. I was plain ol' tired! Many days I felt I was hitting a wall. Sometimes I took a few steps backward on my journey. I might have cheated on my diet or just had a miserable day. It was easy to throw myself a pity party, and I did a couple of times.

But quitting was never an option. Sure, I sometimes felt sorry for myself, but I never allowed it to get to the point where I stopped working hard on my road to getting my health back. It's important to remind yourself that this is a fitness *challenge*. It's not a walk in the park. It's not a vacation. It's not a holiday. It is a challenge and it is hard work.

You are breaking new ground and going places you may not have gone before. You will not be perfect and you will fall down at times, but you must not quit. The worst thing you can do is throw yourself a pity party that never ends. When you indulge in the times where you want to step back and feel sorry for yourself, you are one step away from quitting.

When I had those times, one of my best friends would ask me, "How do you want to be remembered, Amy? Do you want to be a quitter or a winner?" Those were hard words to hear, but I needed to hear them. I wanted my friend to feel sorry for me. I wanted him to say, "Oh, poor Amy. I know you're having a hard time. You deserve to cheat a little. It must be so hard." I'm so glad he never said anything like that.

I know this "Challenge" is tough. Sometimes it feels as though we will never reach our goals. Sometimes we face setbacks. Sometimes it's hard to push ourselves to the next level. Here's some good news. We cannot be defeated if we just stay in the game and don't quit. Tomorrow is another day. Stop feeling sorry for yourself. Get past the momentary setbacks because they are just that—momentary. Get around people who believe in you and who make you a better person. Celebrate all your victories. Even if you just stayed the same and the scale did not budge, at least you didn't gain weight.

You are learning and growing. Bad days and challenges are part of the process. Keep your eyes focused on where you are headed and never give up. If you are tempted to throw yourself a pity party, rip up the invitation. You will get where you want to go, one step at a time. We believe in you. We know you can do it!

Mini-Challenge of the Day

Where do you find strength in tough times? Some people call their friends for encouragement. Others may pray. What is something that you fall back on to give you support? Remember to do that very thing when you are tempted to feel sorry for yourself after a bad day or if you've stumbled on your journey.

____

____

____

Tip of the Day

When you make a healthy salad, don't ruin it by loading it down with high-calorie dressings. Stick with low-calorie and sugar-free dressing alternatives or basic oil and vinegar. I use chunky salsas or specialty mustards such as three-pepper mustard or oil-free ginger dressing.

Meal	Record Your Food & Water Intake for the Day	Calories
1		
2		
3		
4		
5		
	Total Calories	

Fitness Plan

Cardio activity: ______________ Time: ______ Miles: _____

Intensity level (circle one): L M H

Strength training (circle): Lower body Upper body Core

My Thoughts

____

____

____

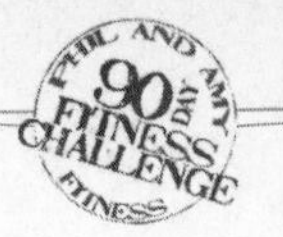

DAY 55—RUN FOR YOUR LIFE

"Great is the man who has not lost his childlike heart."

Mencius, ancient Chinese philosopher

A Note from Amy

One night I needed some extra encouragement before I did a weekend "Fitness Challenge." I texted a friend and asked him to pray for me so that I would have the right things to say to the people coming to our event. The next morning I got this beautiful and profound text from him: "Ask the people this—When is the last time you ran? Ran like you did as a child? That running-on-the-playground kind of run, that running-through-the-hot-summer-sand-into-the-crashing-waves kind of run. Ask them on what day, in what hour, was the last time you ran like that?"

My friend has gone through a major transformation in his life over the last year and he gets it. He understands the importance of living life to the fullest. He sees the need to enjoy and make the most of every moment. He realizes how precious time is, a gift not to be wasted but to be used for a purpose.

When we grow up, we take on heavy responsibilities. We are not as carefree as we once were as children. Now, I understand that we adults cannot act like children most of the time, but I believe there are times when we need to capture that inner child, that little boy or girl inside each of us that loves to be active and have fun and enjoy life.

Think about what you were like as a child. Did you love to play? Did you love to run around the playground? Did you love to chase your friends or your pet? Did you love to have races that you began by saying, "Last one to the ______ is a rotten egg?" I've got a secret to share with you. If you are active and move your body in some way each day, you will scrape away the layers and find that inner child. Finding that carefree, spirited, and enthusiastic little boy or girl can fuel your journey to success and can help you reach your goals.

Here's something else to think about. You are engaged in this challenge today because you have decided to start the race to save your life. In both a figurative and literal sense, you probably started this challenge by walking, taking steps to your goal of a healthier you. Your walk will soon turn into a jog and that jog into a run. You will finally be able to run longer and faster than you ever have. You will finally be able to push through and run past obstacles that have kept you back. You will run as hard and as long as when you were a kid.

Be empowered. Keep running strong. Remember the feelings, hopes, and dreams that you had as a child. Bring some of that inner and younger you to the outside and keep running to save your life.

Mini-Challenge of the Day

Is running a part of your exercise regimen? How fast can you run a mile? How many miles can you run a day? If you run regularly, fantastic. If not, why don't you try running this week? You don't have to run like a marathoner. Just set a goal for one or two miles this week and, when you run, run as though you were a child. It'll feel so good.

Tip of the Day

Get a massage now and then. When you are losing weight and on a workout plan, stress can set in. A massage can get the circulation moving, release your tight muscles, and sometimes even speed up your weight loss.

Meal	Record Your Food & Water Intake for the Day	Calories
1		
2		
3		
4		
5		
	Total Calories	

Fitness Plan

Cardio activity: ____________________ Time: ________ Miles: ______

Intensity level (circle one): L M H

Strength training (circle): Lower body Upper body Core

My Thoughts

____

____

____

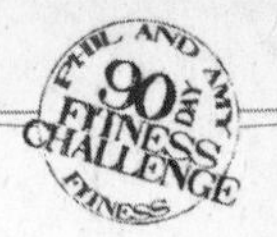

DAY 56—TREASURE IN YOU

*"If you compare yourself to others,
you may become vain and bitter; for always there will
be greater and lesser persons than yourself."*
MAX EHRMANN

A Word from Amy

Do you believe that you have a treasure inside of you? You should, because it's true. We all have something valuable inside of us to give to the world. Even though we may be rough on the outside or seemingly less equipped than others to do great things, we still have greatness inside wanting to come out.

I am guilty of comparing myself to other people. I am sitting in a park as I write this, and occasionally I'll look up and see someone walking by that I envy. I'll think, *I wish my waist was as small as hers,* or *Her hair is gorgeous. I wish mine were like that.* It's silly I know, but I think many of us do this from time to time. Instead of seeing the beauty and wonder of how unique we are, we wish we had something someone else has—whether it's material stuff, talent, abilities, a job, or even a certain body shape.

God has given us everything we need to fulfill the plans He has for us. I can't do what you are called to do, and you can't do what I am called to do. That's why the Bible calls us the body of Christ. We each have a part to play, and God has put in us a specific gift created to bless and help other people. If you never recognize the treasure that you are and you don't value what God has given you, then you may never do the things God has planned for your life.

We need to stop feeling weak or inadequate, looking at what we don't have, and start being empowered by the fact that we are well-equipped to do whatever God wants us to do. After all, it is He who is working in us and fills in the gaps in our lives with His power. As Paul said, "I can do everything through Christ, who gives me strength" (Philippians 4:13).

Be thankful today for the treasure that is in you. The Bible tells us we need to think about things that are pure, lovely, and admirable (Philippians 4:8). When we focus on the good things, it's amazing how they get bigger. The same is true when you focus on the negative. Whatever you focus on gets larger. So the choice is yours as to which one you allow to get larger in your life. Choose the positive. Focus on the treasure that is within you.

Mini-Challenge of the Day

Buy a small journal and make it your "Thankful Journal." Every night before you go to bed, write down five things that you are thankful for. The more you are thankful, the more things come your way that are positive. Anytime you are tempted to look at what you don't have, look at your journal, and you will remember all the wonderful things you have to be thankful for.

Tip of the Day

Keep a calorie counter book with you wherever you go. It will be useful if you are eating out or as you are preparing meals (Phil and I use *The Calorie King Calorie, Fat and Carbohydrate Counter* by Allan Borushek). Over time, you will memorize the calories in the foods you eat most often.

Meal	Record Your Food & Water Intake for the Day	Calories
1		
2		
3		
4		
5		
	Total Calories	

Fitness Plan

Cardio activity: ____________________ Time: ________ Miles: _____

Intensity level (circle one): L M H

Strength training (circle): Lower body Upper body Core

My Thoughts

____

____

____

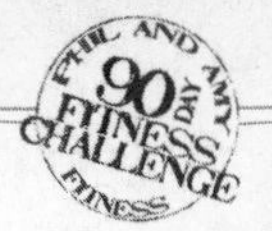

DAY 57—STAY TOUGH TO THE END

"Nothing can stop the man with the right mental attitude from achieving his goal; nothing on earth can help the man with the wrong mental attitude."

Thomas Jefferson

A Note from Phil

I love to watch different kinds of sporting events. It's inspiring to watch amazing athletes who have the mental toughness that gets them through to the finish line (often under a lot of pressure). Michael Jordan used to work miracles in the fourth quarter of his basketball games. Lance Armstrong won the Tour de France bicycle race seven years in a row and also battled cancer. He always knew how to rise to the occasion, year after year. Where does this winner's attitude come from?

First, these athletes set a goal. They worked very hard to reach their goals and never quit. They probably pushed their limits for every workout and practice. They also believed, deep inside, that they could do it. When other people start to think about failing under pressure, these guys think only about victory. Winners push through to the end.

This principle applies to us too. Sometimes that belief in oneself is the last push needed for victory in the home stretch. That kind of mental fortitude is what separates those who succeed and those who quit. But why do many of us give up when we're almost to the finish line?

My friend who is a life coach coaches a famous cyclist. This athlete shared with her that in his opinion his best skill wasn't being a climber. She pressed him further and found that as a child, the cyclist won every race he ever competed in. Most of the races were on the East Coast, where the roads were pretty flat. The championship race one year was in Colorado, and he came in second and felt like he had failed somehow. That one race planted the belief in his mind that his true skills were in only flatland races. His coach, however, helped him through his mental block, and after this discovery he went on to have the best year of his career. It is amazing how just a small change in our mindset can totally alter our outcomes.

We all have self-limiting beliefs or ways that we sabotage our success. The famous athletes you see on TV or read about in the paper are no different than we are. They've just learned to rise above their internal struggles. They choose to focus on the possibilities of winning and success instead of focusing on failure. They keep their mind clear and sharp and never lose sight of the goal.

It's time to power up and get tough. When you want to give up, keep going. When you want to give up this challenge, keep pressing on. You are stronger than you think.

Mini-Challenge of the Day

Plan to finish strong. Think of one area that's causing you to want to quit. What is one way you can prevent yourself from failure in that area? For example, if you always sabotage your success by shortening your workouts, ask yourself why. Then figure out a way that you will not sabotage the remaining weeks of your challenge.

____

____

____

Tip of the Day

Did you know the more prepared a supermarket food is, the more expensive it is? Buying ready-made grilled chicken strips could cost 40 percent more than if you bought chicken breast, grilled it, and cut it into slices yourself. Take the extra time to prepare your food.

Meal	Record Your Food & Water Intake for the Day	Calories
1		
2		
3		
4		
5		
	Total Calories	

Fitness Plan

Cardio activity: ____________________ Time: ________ Miles: ______

Intensity level (circle one): L M H

Strength training (circle): Lower body Upper body Core

My Thoughts

____

____

____

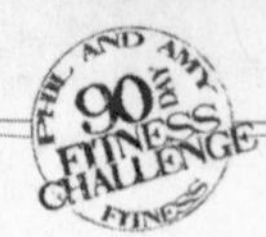

DAY 58—LOSING WEIGHT TOGETHER

"The future is literally in our hands to mold as we like. But we cannot wait until tomorrow. Tomorrow is now."

Eleanor Roosevelt

Jason and Wendy Bauer are a precious couple with a young family who realized they needed to get healthy to be there for their kids. Every time we see them, we are so proud of their accomplishments and that they made their health a priority. Read what Wendy says about their journey.

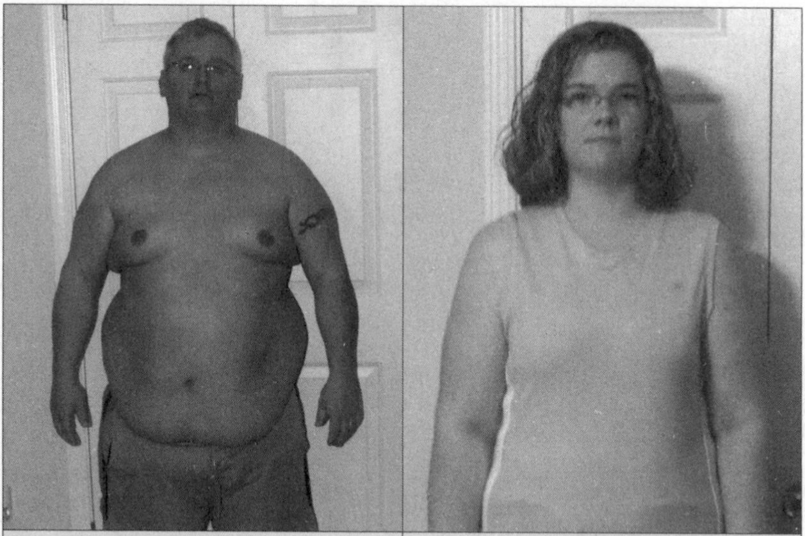

Before	Before
JASON BAUER	**WENDY BAUER**
Weight Loss: 45 lbs.	**Weight Loss: 16 lbs.**

PHOTOS BY JOY M. LOWE

"Before I began the 'Challenge,' I had been working out and following a weight-loss plan. I had successfully lost 25 pounds and then hit a plateau. I needed to lose more weight, and I believed the '90-Day Fitness Challenge' would get me going again. My biggest concern was my husband, Jason. He weighed over 350 pounds, but I didn't know the exact figure because the scale didn't go higher than that. I was scared that I was going to lose the love of my life and the father of our three wonderful kids. I believed the 'Challenge' would make a difference in both our lives.

"To my surprise, Jason was the first to sign up and even started a week earlier than I did. At the weigh-in, he was upset at how much weight he had gained over the years. I thought he would be discouraged and give up before he even began, but he didn't, and I'm so glad for that.

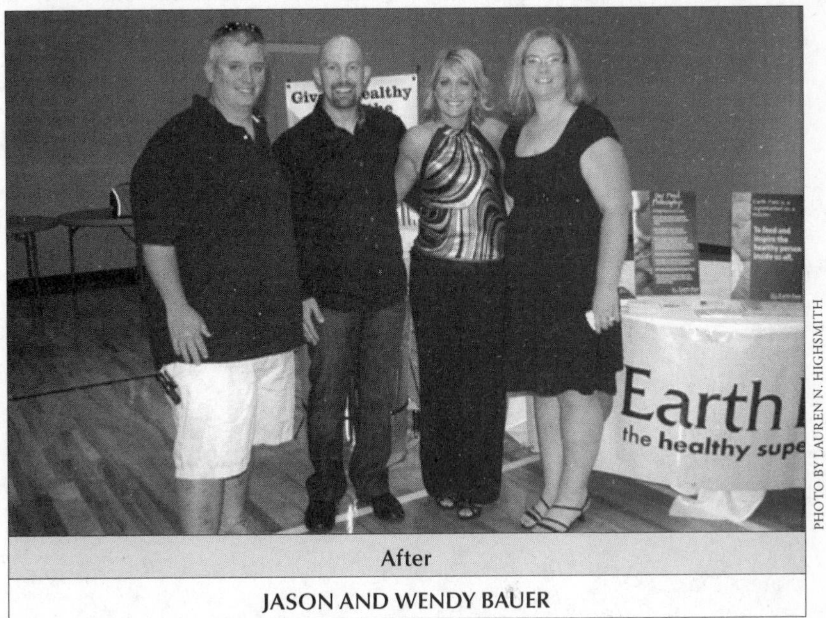

PHOTO BY LAUREN N. HIGHSMITH

After

JASON AND WENDY BAUER

"We both worked together to make all the changes Phil and Amy suggested. We substituted healthy foods for unhealthy foods. We worked out together instead of sitting on the couch. The biggest change is we readjusted our mind-set. We both had a 'can't do it' attitude and didn't realize we had passed that same mentality on to our children. Our new attitude is 'can-do' and positive. We now know we can do anything we put our minds to. Our children have noticed this difference, and they have become more positive too.

"Together Jason and I have lost eighty-five pounds. That's more than our seven-year-old child weighs. In the twelve years we've been together, I have never seen Jason this small. He has gone from a 4X shirt size to 2X and has had to tighten his belt from the second hole to the fifth hole. I went from a size 18 to a 14. We both feel great and are looking better each week."

Mini-Challenge of the Day

Call your spouse, sibling, or loved one and invite him or her to take a walk with you at your local park. Have a great time catching up, appreciating one another, and getting some cardio in.

Tip of the Day

It's always a good idea to eat your chicken without the skin because the skin has the most amount of fat. Also, stick to the chicken breast, which is the leanest part. If you have to choose between dark and white meat, choose the white meat (again, less fat).

Meal	Record Your Food & Water Intake for the Day	Calories
1		
2		
3		
4		
5		
	Total Calories	

Fitness Plan

Cardio activity: ______________________ Time: ________ Miles: ______

Intensity level (circle one): L M H

Strength training (circle): Lower body Upper body Core

My Thoughts

____

____

____

Best Practices:
Eight Best Practices for Success

A few important life themes are crucial for your long-term success. If you can master your attitude, your habits, and keep your focus, you are almost guaranteed success. Learn how to always take care of yourself through all of life's ups and downs.

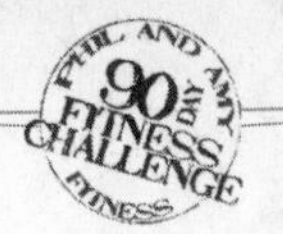

DAY 59—RESPECT

"Self-respect is a question of recognizing that anything worth having has a price."
Joan Didion

A Note from Phil

In college, my friends and I would frequently go to a karaoke lounge. Without fail, we'd see a group of girls on stage belting out "Respect" by Aretha Franklin, and it was always fun to sing along in the crowd.

Thinking about that song made me wonder how much I respected myself over the years. I want to say yes, of course I respected myself. I married a wonderful woman, I have beautiful children, and I'm proud to have a successful career. But I didn't have respect for my body. I didn't take care of it. I didn't feed it well. I didn't give it enough water. I eventually became obese, damaged my joints, and put myself at risk for diabetes and heart disease. Sometimes it's still difficult for me to admit that I had such little respect for my body.

Your thoughts and actions toward yourself and your body are important. When you start to respect your body, the world starts changing for you. Have you ever heard someone say, "Just take care of yourself and everything will fall into place"? I never believed that because I always had to do a million things to make everything fall into place. How could I find time to take care of myself? But after doing just that and getting fit and healthy, a whole new world opened up to me, and everything really did start falling into place—the right place. Loving and respecting yourself will start to bring a whole new perspective on life. You will begin to attract people and opportunities you never thought were possible before.

Recently, Amy and I were eating dinner at a Lebanese restaurant after a busy day. We looked at each other and smiled. I told her how neat it was that we could take some time away for ourselves to enjoy each other's company over a delicious, exotic meal. A year ago, we never even knew this place existed. We would have never thought to look for healthy international cuisine. It's a simple example, but one of the many changes in our lives.

I had to first make the commitment to change. I had to respect and see the value in my body, Only then did my life truly change for the better. Yours can too. Respect yourself.

Mini-Challenge of the Day

Today, reflect on your body and how you take care of yourself. How did you respect and value yourself a year ago? How do you respect yourself today? Has it changed? You can't make permanent lifestyle changes unless you respect yourself.

Tip of the Day

Choose whole fruits over fruit juices. Fruit juice is full of concentrated sugars, and drinking too much juice can cause your blood sugar levels to spike. If you're going to have juice, mix it half-and-half with water. This is how we give juice to our kids too. They quickly got used to the difference, and now, when they drink 100 percent juice, they think it's too sweet.

Meal	Record Your Food & Water Intake for the Day	Calories
1		
2		
3		
4		
5		
	Total Calories	

Fitness Plan

Cardio activity: ______________________ Time: ________ Miles: ______

Intensity level (circle one): L M H

Strength training (circle): Lower body Upper body Core

My Thoughts

____

____

____

DAY 60—ATTITUDE

"When my attitudes are right, there is no barrier too high, no valley too deep, no dream too extreme, no challenge too great for me."
CHARLES R. SWINDOLL

A Note from Phil

My pastor talked about attitude recently in an eight-week sermon series. He used the well-known illustration of viewing a glass as either half-full or half-empty. It's not the glass that tells us which it is; it's how we perceive it. At the time, my pastor was leading our church in a new building program. His wife, pregnant with their fourth child, had been bedridden for most of her pregnancy. He had to take care not only of his congregation, but also his wife and children. Still, he maintained a positive attitude through it all and graciously accepted any help that was offered. He continued to lead, inspire, build, and nurture those around him.

We may not always be able to change the world we see around us, but we can change the way we see the world. Everyone who knows my son Rhett can tell you there is rarely a day when he is not the happiest and most excited person in the room. I watch him and wonder what it must be like to be so carefree. Rhett is happy whether he's coloring or on the computer. He couldn't tell you the difference between one dollar and a million dollars. He doesn't understand it, nor does he care to. To watch the joy he has for the simplest things in life is truly a gift.

Your attitude makes all the difference. Charles Swindoll said it best:

> The longer I live, the more I realize the impact of attitude on life. Attitude, to me, is more important than facts. It is more important than the past, the education, the money, than circumstances, than failure, than successes, than what other people think or say or do. It is more important than appearance, giftedness or skill. It will make or break a company, a church, a home. The remarkable thing is we have a choice every day regarding the attitude we will embrace for that day. We cannot change our past...we cannot change the fact that people will act in a certain way. We cannot change the inevitable. The only thing we can do is play on the one string we have, and that is our attitude. I am convinced that life is 10% what happens to me and 90% of how I react to it.

Mini-Challenge of the Day

Today, reflect on the quote by Charles Swindoll. Attitude will make or break your lifestyle change. Is there an area in your life where your attitude can improve? Make that adjustment today.

Tip of the Day

Reduce stress. I know, so simple yet so hard to do. Eliminating even a little bit of stress does wonders for your health. Get a massage. Sleep a little extra. Take a yoga class. Pray more. Do something to ease your mind and your soul, and better health will follow.

Meal	Record Your Food & Water Intake for the Day	Calories
1		
2		
3		
4		
5		
	Total Calories	

Fitness Plan

Cardio activity: ______________________ Time: ________ Miles: _____

Intensity level (circle one): L M H

Strength training (circle): Lower body Upper body Core

My Thoughts

____

____

____

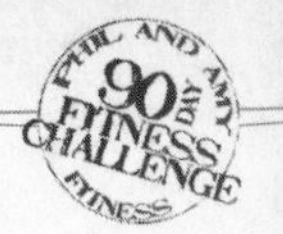

DAY 61—RICE

"Take care of your body.
It's the only place you have to live."
Jim Rohn

A Word from Amy

I was blessed during my weight-loss process on the ranch that I never got a sports injury, though I was sore many times. It's embarrassing to admit, but sometimes I thought my peers who complained about their ailments were just whiners. Eventually I came to understand what they were going through.

A few weeks ago, I noticed my knee hurt when I ran. So I stopped running and started walking on a treadmill at a higher incline. My knee felt better after that change. Then I was involved in a fitness project, and I had to run two miles for a physical training test. My knee felt as if it were on fire, but I ran through the pain. The next day, I couldn't run at all. It was scary not knowing exactly what was wrong with my knee. Did I seriously hurt it? Would I ever be able to run again?

I went to a physical therapist, and he told me I had "runner's knee." It's a common problem with runners, and he prescribed strengthening exercises to alleviate my condition. He also suggested using RICE three times a day to reduce the pain and inflammation—*rest* the injury, *ice* it, apply a *compress* by wrapping it, and then *elevate* the leg. It worked!

I was relieved to get the professional advice I needed and was glad I didn't have to stop running forever. I just had to take better care of myself. Now I make sure to warm up before I exercise, and every now and then I put an ice pack on my knee even if it doesn't hurt.

Most people on a weight-loss journey, especially if they are working out every day, will experience an injury at some point. You should always seek the advice of a doctor or therapist if you have unusual pain. The longer you wait, the greater the chances the temporary injury could turn into a permanent one. The important thing is to not let your injuries stop you from your journey. Here are a few tips to prevent this from happening:

- Stretch before and after your workout.
- Use supports or wraps on areas of your body that are especially weak or painful.

- Spend ten minutes in a sauna after a workout to reduce soreness the next day.
- Wear properly fitted sneakers.
- Pay attention. Watch where you're stepping. Instead of trying to carry ten bags of groceries up the stairs so you have to make only one trip, be safe and take two trips instead.
- When you are lifting weights, use proper form.

Mini-Challenge of the Day

RICE is one of the most important things you should know to keep yourself injury-free. Refresh your memory for what each letter stands for and write it down below.

R: ____________________

I: ____________________

C: ____________________

E: ____________________

If your pain or swelling doesn't decrease in forty-eight hours, see a doctor.

Tip of the Day

Did you know that garlic is good for you? According to studies published in the *American Journal of Clinical Nutrition*, garlic is good not only for your heart, it may also help prevent stomach and colon cancers. Aim to eat five cloves of raw or cooked garlic a week.

Meal	Record Your Food & Water Intake for the Day	Calories
1		
2		
3		
4		
5		
	Total Calories	

Fitness Plan

Cardio activity: ______________________ Time: ________ Miles: _____

Intensity level (circle one): L M H

Strength training (circle): Lower body Upper body Core

My Thoughts

____

____

____

DAY 62—CONSISTENCY

"At all times it is better to have a method."
Mark Caine

A Note from Phil

There is real power in consistency. Think about this. If you worked out one day per year, how would your body look? What if you worked out once a month? Your body would probably still look the same. But what if you worked out every single day for one year? Your body would look amazing, and you would feel incredible. All the positive daily habits and routines we are teaching you, if applied consistently, will help you achieve incredible results. The key is consistency. If you do the right thing all or most of the time, you will break through and win.

When I was on my weight-loss journey, I wished I saw results faster. It was easy to get discouraged about the minor ups and downs. But I regularly applied the tips and techniques that I was taught, despite how I felt. I never stopped. I took my little notebook with me everywhere to write in my food journal. I worked out every day. I drank the water my body needed. I prepared all my foods on the weekends, even if I was tired. It wasn't easy, but it was simple.

Some days I went to the gym and told my trainer, D.J., I didn't feel like working out that day. He would tell me to get on the treadmill anyway, and then ask me to talk about my feelings. It was an interesting technique. I was complaining about not wanting to do something while I was doing it. Without fail, at the end of the workout, I felt great and my attitude had changed for the better.

Most people become frustrated and quit, especially when they hit a plateau. When you get to that dreaded place, change things up. Vary the intensity of your workouts or change some of the foods you're eating. If you give up and stop doing what you know you need to be doing, you'll never break through to the next level.

You need to consistently do the right things. This must be a nonnegotiable for you. Stay in the game, and I promise you will see results. Persistence overcomes resistance!

Mini-Challenge of the Day

Look at any area that you need to be more consistent. Are you drinking enough water every day? Are you eating the right meals every day? Are you getting the right exercise every day? Are you applying the good habits we are teaching you every day? If you're going to win, you are going to have to be consistent.

Tip of the Day

Soup is one of the most affordable and delicious meals to make. Buy vegetables on sale. Buy the cheaper chicken or beef parts used for soup. Throw in some pasta for texture. Boil, simmer for two hours, and you'll have a delicious and hearty meal. Freeze the soup in smaller containers for the week.

Meal	Record Your Food & Water Intake for the Day	Calories
1		
2		
3		
4		
5		
	Total Calories	

Fitness Plan

Cardio activity: ______________________ Time: ________ Miles: ______

Intensity level (circle one): L M H

Strength training (circle): Lower body Upper body Core

My Thoughts

____

____

____

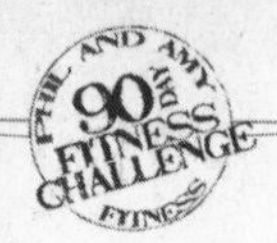

DAY 63—LOSE THE CRUTCH

"Courage is the power to let go of the familiar."
RAYMOND LINDQUIST

A Note from Phil

Does a pastry care about you? Do cookies love you? Will it make you feel better if you finish a whole bottle of wine? No. No. And no. In the past, I made poor choices by abusing food and alcohol. I misused those things to cover up my real problems.

I call them crutches. Many of us have them. A crutch can be food, alcohol, cigarettes, video games, TV—it makes no difference. Crutches temporarily remove you from reality so you don't have to deal with your issues. But your problems are still there. They aren't going anywhere. All your crutch is doing is keeping you another day away from reaching your dreams.

Crutches are so popular and tempting because they do numb pain for a time. It's pleasurable to indulge in a few glasses of wine or your favorite cake. All your problems seem to fade away. Crutches also give you a sense of security. It feels comforting to eat a pint of ice cream at night. But how does it feel the next morning? Does it feel comforting and nurturing? No, I don't think so. Instead, you probably feel guilty and bloated.

When you take away the crutch of food, you have to make a choice. Do you finally deal with the issues you've been running from or do you go back to your old ways? When you decide to make powerful change in your life, internal problems will come up. We all have our issues, but we don't have to be afraid of them. They are simply opportunities God gives us to help strengthen us. As tough as it is, we must search inside ourselves and make the choice to better ourselves. We need to be honest and ask God, who is always there for us, to help us through the pain.

Let's face it. There might be times when you cannot deal with things in that moment. You may have to wait until later to work through it. When pressure comes, take a minute. Relax. Ask yourself what you need. Do you need to exercise? Do you need to be alone? Do you need to talk to someone? A more positive response is always available. There is always a way to resolve the problem without going back to your crutch.

Lose the crutch. Face yourself, and you will become a stronger person. You can do it.

Mini-Challenge of the Day

Write down one of your crutches. What is one thing you still feel like going back to when you don't want to deal with an issue? Make a choice today that you will not return to your crutch no matter what happens today.

____

____

____

Tip of the Day

Don't forget to exercise your abdominals. Spend at least five minutes doing crunches after each weight routine. If there is an abdominal or core class at the gym, go at least once. It will give you great ideas of the different ways to work your abs.

Meal	Record Your Food & Water Intake for the Day	Calories
1		
2		
3		
4		
5		
	Total Calories	

Fitness Plan

Cardio activity: ________________ Time: _______ Miles: _____

Intensity level (circle one): L M H

Strength training (circle): Lower body Upper body Core

My Thoughts

____

____

____

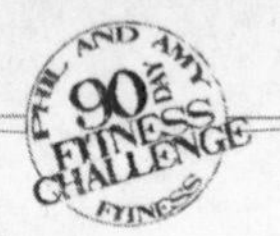

DAY 64—FOCUS

"Our thoughts create our reality—where we put our focus is the direction we tend to go."
PETER MCWILLIAMS

A Note from Phil

When you started the "90-Day Fitness Challenge," you set your focus and wrote down your goals (see appendix A). When we were on the ranch, we also set goals. Our goal was to lose as much weight as possible and win the competition. Even after we were sent home, we were always working toward that goal and the prize for the most weight lost. While I was in competition mode, I was focused. I read my goals daily and worked hard to meet them.

I ultimately achieved them by losing a tremendous amount of weight and completely changing my lifestyle. The week after the season finale of the show, I was able to relax. There was no final weigh-in to work toward, so a bit of the pressure was off. Then the trouble began. Although I had the support of the show and my *Biggest Loser* peers, I started drifting along like a boat without an anchor. With the competition aspect over, I had no more direction. I never realized that when I reached the maintenance stage, I would feel so lost. Was this all there was? Just eating a few meals and working out every day? I had lost the thrill and the excitement of the health journey. I had lost my focus.

That happens to many of us. We set out on a journey, and we either make it or we don't. Along the way, all of us will lose, or at least shift, our focus and feel unguided. It's then we have to remember what will keep us on track. For me, I realized that I love challenges. I need to have a goal, a deadline, or a finish line. I thrive on excitement and the pressures of working toward an end result.

When the competition was over, I was just going through the motions. I needed to get my energy back, so I called up a good friend, and we decided we would run the next half-marathon in my town. That was enough for me to put a plan together, and we trained for the next few weeks with that focus in mind. It gave me the motivation to continue my healthy lifestyle, and I also bonded with a good friend.

When the "90-Day Fitness Challenge" is over, don't let your life coast along. If you're not careful, old habits will start creeping back. Your pants will get a bit tighter, and you'll wonder what on earth is happening?. What's happening is that you lost your focus.

It doesn't matter what your next goal is after this "Challenge." Just be sure to create one. It will keep you focused and moving forward. When you make it your mission to keep your life full of positive goals, your life becomes so much more exciting.

Mini-Challenge of the Day

Today, think about your next focus. What is the next active goal that interests you after you complete the "Challenge"? Write it down. It could be hiking up the tallest mountain in your state, attending martial arts classes, or joining a competitive adult swim league. The possibilities are endless!

___

___

___

___

Tip of the Day

Get a small rice cooker. They can be pricey ($150 average), but they're a worthwhile investment. Your rice will come out perfectly, and it will save you time in the kitchen. This piece of cookware makes rice, broths, and porridge. I've put some chicken and vegetables in with the rice to steam. Ten minutes later, I have a few meals ready for the week. Instead of water, use low-sodium chicken broth to add extra flavor.

Meal	Record Your Food & Water Intake for the Day	Calories
1		
2		
3		
4		
5		
	Total Calories	

Fitness Plan

Cardio activity: ______________________ Time: ________ Miles: ______

Intensity level (circle one): L M H

Strength training (circle): Lower body Upper body Core

My Thoughts

____

____

____

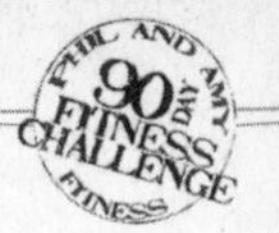

DAY 65—CHOOSE CHANGE

"The only constant is change."
Heraclitus

A Note from Phil

Change is inevitable. Your life today will be different than your life a year from now.

In May 2008, I was fat. In December that same year, I was thin. When I was fat, I was the life of the party and made everyone laugh. Just seven months later, I wasn't sure who I was. I lost weight faster than my mind could keep up. I was doing things I had never done before and eating things I had never eaten before. I was making all the changes that I needed. J.D. Roth, narrator and executive producer of *The Biggest Loser,* had told us, "You just have to embrace the process." That is easier said than done.

Several times along the way, my middle son, Pearson, looked at me and said, "Daddy, you don't look very happy. I'm worried about you." He wanted to rescue me from my pain, but the truth was, he couldn't help me. I had to work through my stuff the best way I knew how. Many times I was smiling on the outside, but I was sad on the inside. Other times I just felt lost. After forty years of being a certain way, I was being challenged on every level. People related to me differently than before. I suddenly felt insecure in areas I had felt secure before.

During those rough months, I believe I was going through a mourning process for the old me, while discovering and learning to love the new me. It's as though I had to pass from one life to the next. It was dark and unfamiliar territory, but one day, the sun came out. Rediscovering myself was a growth process, not a one-time event.

I love the new me. I have reinvented my life. I no longer feel I need to be the center of attention. Every day I look forward to doing new things. Change is good. Embrace the process and the different changes that come with weight loss. Don't go back to your old habits even though it may be more comfortable. It's not worth it. Choose change, not comfort.

Mini-Challenge of the Day

Reflect on and pray this prayer: "God, it's hard, but I choose to embrace all the changes in my life. I know that You are with me every step of the way.

I may not always feel happy and secure, but I am depending on You for help and strength. I choose to honor the changes in my life and keep the focus on my health instead of running back to what feels comforting. You are my comfort."

Tip of the Day

Going out socially is a great way to network and meet people, but how do you balance health, eating out, and your social life? Make time to network over breakfast. It's easier to eat healthy at breakfast and cheaper too.

Meal	Record Your Food & Water Intake for the Day	Calories
1		
2		
3		
4		
5		
	Total Calories	

Fitness Plan

Cardio activity: ______________________ Time: ________ Miles: ______

Intensity level (circle one): L M H

Strength training (circle): Lower body Upper body Core

My Thoughts

____

____

____

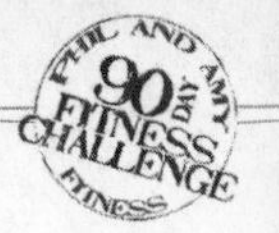

DAY 66—**SUBSTITUTE**

"Cultivate only the habits that you are willing should master you."
Elbert Hubbard

A Note from Phil

One of my favorite books is *See You at the Top* by Zig Ziglar. In one of the chapters, he talks about the importance of habits. Did you know that you can't just eliminate habits? You have to substitute a good habit for a bad one. For example, it's very difficult to wake up one day and tell yourself you're never going to eat sugar again. Your mind won't know how to deal with that void. Tell yourself that instead of eating sugar, you're going to replace it with fruits and natural sweeteners such as Stevia. It's much easier for the mind and body to accept substitutes than it is to hear the word *no*. Remember, you want to set yourself up for success, not failure.

I used to live a sedentary life. When I wasn't working, I was a couch potato. It was my idea of relaxation. I was too tired to spend time with the kids, and if I did, we spent it watching TV. After being on the ranch and changing my habits, I knew the coach-potato lifestyle couldn't be for me anymore. I didn't just tell myself to stop lying on the couch watching TV; I had to think of substitutes. So I gave myself some options. After work I could go to the gym, do an activity with my family, or take my wife out to dinner (or do all three!).

You know what happened? I got closer to my boys, I continued to stay fit and healthy, and I found time to recreate romance in my marriage. My life improved. After a while, I didn't miss vegging out on the couch. I was too busy living a great life.

Keep your focus on your new habits. When you do this, the old habits will begin to fade away. One more thing: be patient. Take your time and don't try to change all your bad habits at once. Before you know it, your life will be full of healthy habits and you will experience a *new* life.

Mini-Challenge of the Day

1. Make a list of the things you do that are not healthy, can be addictive, do not serve your higher purpose, and that you don't feel good about.
2. Circle the top two bad habits you want to change.

3. Think of good substitutes. What can you do that is healthy in the place of these two bad habits?
4. Start with the first habit today. Make that change. And take a look at this page every now and then to remind you of what you need to do.

____

____

____

____

Tip of the Day

Supermarkets usually discount their meats up to 60 percent when they are close to their expiration date. Take advantage of these deals. The meat is still fresh, so buy a few pounds extra to store in the freezer.

Meal	Record Your Food & Water Intake for the Day	Calories
1		
2		
3		
4		
5		
	Total Calories	

Fitness Plan

Cardio activity: ____________________ Time: ________ Miles: _____

Intensity level (circle one): L M H

Strength training (circle): Lower body Upper body Core

My Thoughts

____

____

____

DAY 67—EXCITED FOR A NEW LIFE

"Growth is the only evidence of life."

John Henry Newman, *Apologia Pro Vita Sua* (1864)

Jimmy and Kathleen Bacon are always smiling. Their love for each other is obvious and the way they worked together on the "Challenge" is inspiring. They started exercising with our personal trainer, D.J. Jordan, and they continue to do great. Read what Kathleen has to say.

PHOTO BY EMILY HAYNES

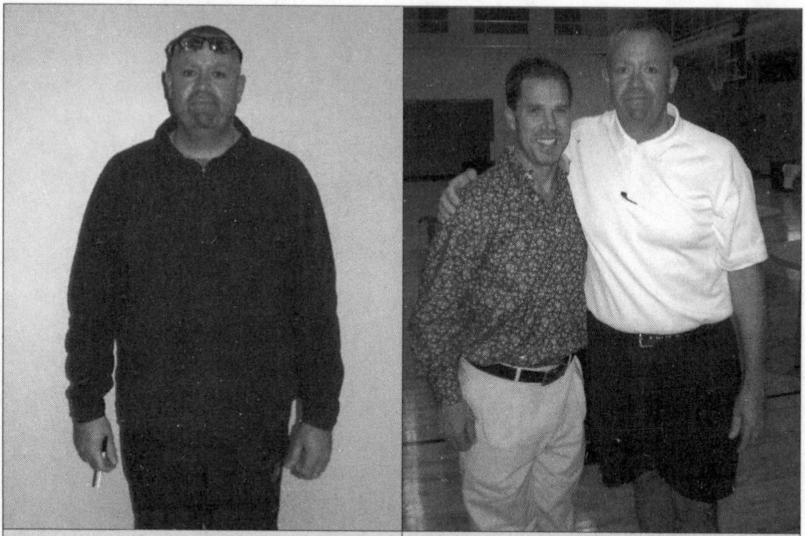

PHOTO BY KATHLEEN BACON

Before	After
JIMMY BACON	
Weight Loss: 27 lbs.	

"Two and a half years ago, after years of not taking care of myself, I was at my highest weight and desperate enough that I was preparing for gastric bypass surgery. I was devastated to find out that my insurance would not cover the procedure. I didn't have a choice but to try to lose weight on my own. I worked with my doctor, joined a weight-loss program, and started exercising. I lost sixty pounds and felt pretty good, but I was only on a diet; I had not truly changed my lifestyle. I would go to the program meetings on Saturday mornings and weigh in, only to binge the rest of the weekend. I eventually got real sick and was diagnosed with fibromyalgia. I gained back forty pounds and was miserable every day.

"I heard about the '90-Day Fitness Challenge' through a friend. I decided to give it a try and work on losing the weight I gained back. This challenge has helped me to make permanent lifestyle changes. It's so different this time. I actually enjoy eating healthy and love to exercise (in the past, I hated any and all physical activity). My life has never been better. I lost weight and my cholesterol dropped from 213 to 139 and my triglycerides from 275 to 115. I look forward to continuing on with more weight loss, better health, and all the things my husband, Jimmy, and I will be able to do together.

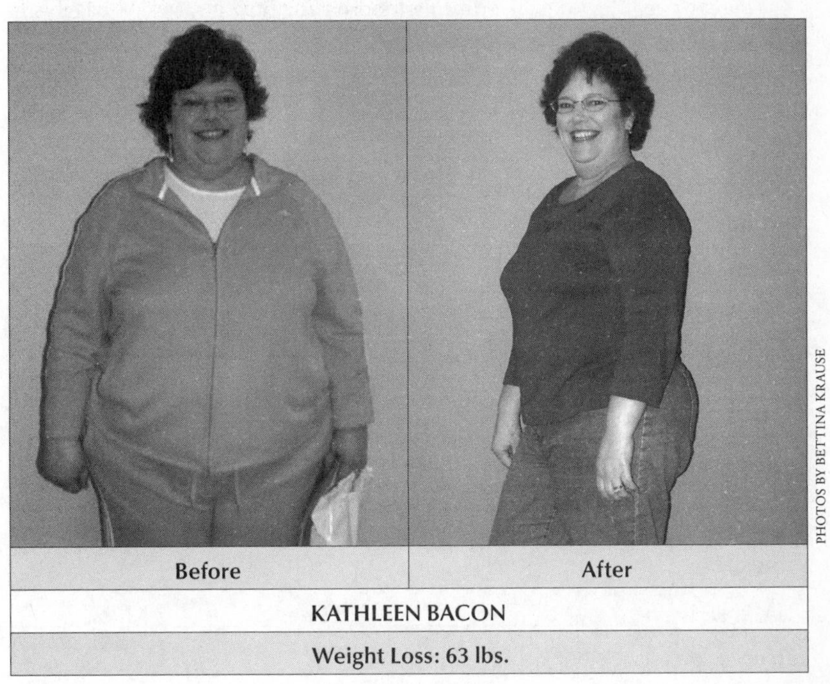

Before	After
KATHLEEN BACON	
Weight Loss: 63 lbs.	

PHOTOS BY BETTINA KRAUSE

"Jimmy decided to join the 'Challenge' with me to get healthier and to be my support. He feels great and enjoys daily exercise at the gym. He went from not working out at all to working out six days a week, sometimes even twice a day. His weight loss happened so quickly that his clothes look like they are falling off him. His cholesterol dropped from 210 to 174 and his triglycerides from 155 to 88.

"D.J. Jordan, my personal trainer, has been instrumental in my success. He started out as a complete stranger, and now I am accountable to him for everything I do every day. And if it weren't for Phil and Amy, I don't know where I would be today."

Mini-Challenge of the Day

Spend extra time stretching after your workout. Add fifteen seconds to every stretch. Stretch more deeply than you ever thought you could. Your body will thank you.

Tip of the Day

You can't tell how much sodium a food has by how it tastes. A bagel isn't very salty, is it? But guess what? An oat-bran bagel has 451 mg of sodium. The best way to know how much sodium a food has is to read the nutrition label.

Meal	Record Your Food & Water Intake for the Day	Calories
1		
2		
3		
4		
5		
	Total Calories	

Fitness Plan

Cardio activity: ______________________ Time: ________ Miles: ______

Intensity level (circle one): L M H

Strength training (circle): Lower body Upper body Core

My Thoughts

____

____

____

Digging Deeper: Beyond Just Dieting and Exercising

The path to achieving your goals isn't perfect. It's time for a reality check into the common pitfalls and struggles as we journey closer to the end of the "Challenge." Now is the time to face your fears, dig even deeper emotionally, and embrace your metamorphosis.

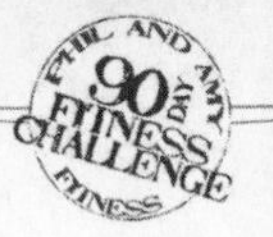

DAY 68—UNWELCOME CHANGES

"Nobody can go back and start a new beginning,
but anyone can start today and make a new ending."
Maria Robinson

A Word from Amy

When I first started watching *The Biggest Loser*, I remember thinking that the contestants must have the most carefree lives once they lost the weight. I imagined they would come home to a better job, a better relationship, a better life, and the world would embrace their success. When I got back from the ranch, I found that wasn't the case at all. Although being on the show has been one of the most amazing opportunities of my life, there were some changes I didn't expect to experience when I got home.

Losing weight is not just about the physical body. It involves emotional issues, hormone fluctuations, and a mental readjustment. The overweight woman who always dreamed of fitting into a size 8 dress finally reaches her goal. When she puts on that dress, instead of excitement and exhilaration, she feels uncomfortable. She doesn't know how to act, how to carry herself, and what to do with all the admiring glances she gets. Her changes have pushed her outside her comfort zone. She has to learn how to adjust her mindset with her new reality.

What about your friends, family, and coworkers? How are they going to react to your weight loss? You might be surprised at how differently others see the new you. They may not know how to act around you. Some will truly be happy for your success, and others might be jealous. I've found that people sometimes like it when you are overweight because it makes them feel better about themselves. I had one friend (I admire her honesty) who told me she was comfortable being around me when I was fat because then she was not the fattest person in the room. Now that I was thin, I was no longer her mental confidence booster.

Another unwelcome change was that it took a while before my mind adjusted to my new size. It didn't happen overnight. I had to take pictures of myself next to people before I could gauge what size I was. Though I had lost the weight and was a size 4, I still saw myself as overweight. Logically, I knew that I was small, but a part of me just didn't believe it. Sometimes I still battle with seeing "fat Amy" in the mirror.

Dealing with the aftermath of your weight loss is a difficult and emotional process. It might force you to face some things you had kept buried. You might have to face unresolved anger or forgive people from your past. After you lose weight, life might not turn out exactly as you imagined it would. Since you are going to be successful in this journey, you need to be aware of the challenges along the way. Be ready for anything.

Mini-Challenge of the Day

We are approaching the end of the "Challenge." What is one thing that hasn't turned out quite the way you expected? Connect with someone who has lost a great deal of weight. Have them share with you a challenge they've had. Learn from their experience so that you are better equipped to handle the unexpected events that will come up in your life.

Tip of the Day

One pound of fat is equivalent to 3500 calories. You will need to burn that amount to lose one pound. If you cut out just 500 calories from your diet per day, you will lose one pound per week.

Meal	Record Your Food & Water Intake for the Day	Calories
1		
2		
3		
4		
5		
	Total Calories	

Fitness Plan

Cardio activity: ____________________ Time: ________ Miles: ______

Intensity level (circle one): L M H

Strength training (circle): Lower body Upper body Core

My Thoughts

____

____

____

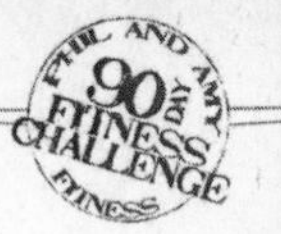

DAY 69—**FEAR FACTOR**

"The only thing we have to fear is fear itself."
FRANKLIN D. ROOSEVELT

A Word from Amy

Have you ever wondered why so many times in the Bible God tells someone to "fear not"? Do you think maybe it's because He knew how important that message is and that we would always need to be reminded of it?

Fear is in the air. There's no doubt about that. There is more fear than ever thanks to the onslaught of news coverage twenty-four hours a day, most of it negative—a global economic crisis, serious environmental issues, higher rates of cancer than in the past, and the usual murders, typhoons, and earthquakes. I don't watch the news anymore because I don't want to be consumed by the negative and scary information being reported.

There are a lot of things we can be afraid of, but all is not lost. There is hope. The best part of trusting in God is knowing that everything is going to work out the way it's supposed to. The Bible tells us that the steps of a good man are ordered by the Lord (Psalm 37:23). This verse has given me much comfort over the years. If I trust God and do the right thing, then He will direct my path. Through Him, I will fulfill my purpose and destiny. This verse gives me the permission to mentally relax.

When I speak in public, I see such a sense of urgency and fear in the eyes of many. I know that look because I've been in their shoes. They feel as if they are running against an invisible hourglass, and they are losing the race. That builds a lot of internal pressure to do more and be more. That anxiety just leads us straight to the fridge to shake away our fears with food.

I've read that there are over a hundred instances in the Bible where we are told not to fear. That's a lot of "fear nots"! Any fear you have will only hold you back. It could be big fears over your financial security or the welfare of your family. It could even be fears of being thin or being afraid of changes you'll have to make on this transformational journey. It's time to let go of fear and trust in God.

Mini-Challenge of the Day

Today, reflect on a fear that might be stopping you in your tracks. If you aren't sure where to start, think about something that you always sabotage.

For example, if you are constantly yo-yo dieting, chances are some fear has not been addressed.

____

____

____

Tip of the Day

Contestants on the show wear what look like black armbands. Those are Bodybuggs used to measure calories. You wear the band on your arm all day, and it measures the number of calories you burn. Once you know how many calories you burn in a day, then you know how many calories you need to limit yourself to to lose weight. You may want to invest in a Bodybugg. Check them out at www.bodybugg.com.

Meal	Record Your Food & Water Intake for the Day	Calories
1		
2		
3		
4		
5		
	Total Calories	

Fitness Plan

Cardio activity: ____________________ Time: ________ Miles: ______

Intensity level (circle one): L M H

Strength training (circle): Lower body Upper body Core

My Thoughts

____

____

____

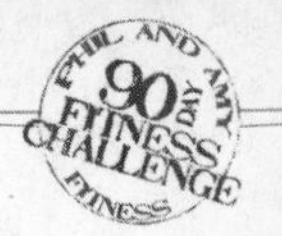

DAY 70—REALITY CHECK

"Reality is something you rise above."
LIZA MINNELLI, ACTRESS AND SINGER

A Word from Amy

When I was dealing with the initial blow of Rhett's diagnosis of autism, one of the predominant questions I had was whether he would be able to live on his own when he grew up. I still do not have the answer to that question. At this point, there is no cure for autism. No one knows what therapies will be available in the years to come. Phil and I have to be prepared that Rhett may live with us for the rest of our lives. This is our reality check.

Coming to terms with that reality early on in Rhett's life made me think about my weight. If my life were cut short because of complications with my weight, then who would be there for Rhett? If I was debilitated, even temporarily, from a heart attack or stroke, who would care for Rhett? Phil was asking these sobering questions too. Those questions were a major motivating factor in my decision to begin this journey toward health.

What about you? What is your reality check? What is motivating you to take a good look at making life changes? Maybe you want to get married. Maybe you want to start a family. Maybe you have recently received a negative report from your doctor. Maybe you are a mom who has no energy left for your children. Maybe you are a dad who is tired of watching your kids play because you don't have the stamina to join them. Or maybe you just want to know that for once in your life, you look pretty darn good. We all have different reasons for wanting to lose weight. Be sure to use your reason to motivate you toward better health.

My kids were the biggest influencers initially in helping me commit to weight loss. As I noticed Phil losing weight as well, I pushed myself even more because I wanted to share the journey with him. Two years later, I've learned to value myself and my health. I've gotten used to feeling good after every workout and loving the way my body looks. Maintaining this lifestyle is a gift to me.

The first place I had to start was facing reality. Now I am confident that unless God has different plans for me, I will be around for my husband and my kids for a long, long time. Use your reality checks to keep you committed to the "Challenge" even when times get tough. You are doing a tremendous job so far. Keep the momentum going!

Mini-Challenge of the Day

At the start of this "Challenge," what was your motivation to make this investment to change your life? What is the reality that will happen if you don't make these changes? This might be something you need to refocus on as you continue toward the finish line.

____

____

____

Tip of the Day

The American College of Sports Medicine recommends that women eat a minimum of 1200 calories a day; for men it's 1500. Eating fewer calories will slow down your metabolism as your body believes it's starving. This is counter-productive to long-term weight loss. So don't cut your calories too much.

Meal	Record Your Food & Water Intake for the Day	Calories
1		
2		
3		
4		
5		
	Total Calories	

Fitness Plan

Cardio activity: ____________________ Time: ________ Miles: ______

Intensity level (circle one): L M H

Strength training (circle): Lower body Upper body Core

My Thoughts

____

____

____

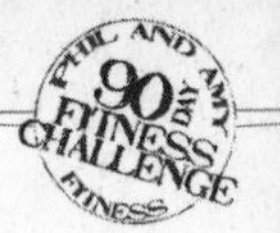

DAY 71—RAIN MAN

"If there is no struggle, there is no progress."
FREDERICK DOUGLASS

A Word from Amy

How many of you have seen the 1988 movie *Rain Man* starring Dustin Hoffman (playing Raymond Babbitt) and Tom Cruise (playing Charlie Babbitt)? It's an exceptional film about two brothers, one of whom is an adult with autism. Hoffman accurately portrays how autistic people are drawn toward routine and lose all control when that routine is broken. For example, Raymond has to go to bed at the same time every night, buy his underwear from a particular Kmart in Cincinnati, and watch particular TV shows at the same time every day. If not, he throws a terrible tantrum.

We see this kind of behavior a lot with Rhett. His current interest is the drive-thru window of fast-food restaurants. He draws pictures of them, looks for videos about them on YouTube, acts like a cashier at the window, and has even turned our kitchen into his personal drive-thru. If we tell him to stop, he'll throw a fit. He gets some type of comfort from the drive-thru scenario, so we let him indulge in that obsession.

A lot of people exhibit similar behavior. It may not be as dramatic as Rhett's or Raymond's, but it's just as powerful. So many folks tell me they can't lose weight because healthy food is too expensive, or they can't give up a certain food, or they were raised eating fried food and they can't break the habit. All these comments suggest an underlying routine or a comfort zone that they aren't willing to leave behind.

I was raised with some terrible eating habits. Food was a source of entertainment and comfort. When I arrived on the ranch, I was amazed to find myself kicking and screaming on the inside, even though I was there to make changes I wanted to make. This big baby inside of me was used to doing whatever it wanted, and it didn't like to be told what to do. My routine was being challenged, and I had to make a choice. I had to tell that tantrum-throwing baby no. I had to be willing to change my habits.

We all have choices to make. You can let your inner food-child run wild, or you can rein her in, one step at a time. It's a choice. You are an adult and you can take charge of your life. Does it get easier? Yes. It gets easier every time you make the right decision for your health. Remember that you have the power to change because you have the power to choose. Choose to be healthy, choose to stay the course, and choose to never give up.

Mini-Challenge of the Day

Is there any part of this journey that you are still kicking and screaming about and refusing to go with the new plan? Write it down. Take a moment to reflect on what exactly you do not want to let go of or believe you can't let go of. If it is a habit that doesn't serve you, you have to let it go to be successful in your challenge. Today, surrender this to God.

____

____

____

Tip of the Day

Chew sugar-free gum in the middle of the afternoon instead of reaching for that high-calorie snack. It will keep your mouth busy, you will feel refreshed, and your teeth will be cleaner. We always make sure to have a pack of gum with us, just in case we need the extra boost during the day.

Meal	Record Your Food & Water Intake for the Day	Calories
1		
2		
3		
4		
5		
	Total Calories	

Fitness Plan

Cardio activity: ____________________ Time: ________ Miles: ______

Intensity level (circle one): L M H

Strength training (circle): Lower body Upper body Core

My Thoughts

____

____

____

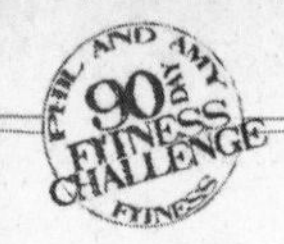

DAY 72—METAMORPHOSIS

"The phoenix hope, can wing her way through the desert skies, and still defying fortune's spite; revive from ashes and rise."

MIGUEL DE CERVANTES SAAVEDRA

A Note from Phil

It's worth repeating—this "Challenge" is about more than just weight loss. It's about your mind, body, and soul. Think about true transformation as an onion; there are many layers to your metamorphosis. Just when you think you've reached a goal (whether you met your weekly weight-loss numbers or completed that difficult workout), you will find another issue, challenge, or test that you must endure. You need to go through all the different layers to truly transform yourself from the inside out.

A few years ago, within the span of twelve months, my business failed, we bought a foreclosure that became a money pit, and our youngest son was diagnosed with autism. During that time, I felt as if God had abandoned me. Even worse, I thought He was punishing me for something I had done. Looking back, I know those experiences were trials by fire so that I could emerge a stronger and more patient man. But when I emerged out of each situation a better person, another challenge awaited me. I needed to go through a few more layers of change.

Being on the show and undergoing that extreme change was a huge test. Would I be able to conquer the body that had held me back for so long? Would I be strong enough to withstand the physical and mental demands of serious change in front of millions of people? My trainer showed me that the same strength I used to deal with the other challenges in my life is the same strength I could use to conquer my weight issue. There and then I realized my weight problem was not about my lack of willpower. It was about using food to comfort the areas where I felt weak. I had to realize that I was strong. Not just in one area, but in all areas. If I could conquer one area, I could conquer them all.

You are undergoing a metamorphosis. Find the strength you've used to succeed in other areas in your life and use it to work on your health and body. It is going to make you a much stronger person.

Mini-Challenge of the Day

Sometimes it's hard for us to find our own strengths (especially if we are used to looking only at our faults). Talk to your best friend, your spouse, or a family member. Ask them to tell you about three areas of your life where they have seen your strength. It could be something you overcame, a competition you won, or just something you succeeded in. Reflect on those situations and draw on that same strength to believe you can succeed on this challenge.

Tip of the Day

A great appetizer at an Asian restaurant is edamame, steamed soybeans in a pod. They're delicious and very healthy for you. You can even buy them in bulk and make them at home. Just put them in the microwave to heat them up, sprinkle on a little low-sodium salt or salt substitute, and enjoy.

Meal	Record Your Food & Water Intake for the Day	Calories
1		
2		
3		
4		
5		
	Total Calories	

Fitness Plan

Cardio activity: ______________________ Time: ________ Miles: ______

Intensity level (circle one): L M H

Strength training (circle): Lower body Upper body Core

My Thoughts

___

___

___

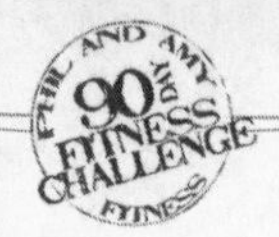

DAY 73—PEARL OF GREAT PRICE

"Again, the kingdom of heaven
is like a merchant looking for fine pearls.
When he found one of great value, he went away
and sold everything he had and bought it."
JESUS (MATTHEW 13:45-46)

A Word from Amy

It's a good idea to periodically evaluate our priorities. Too often I notice how people will say their priority is one thing, but how they live does not reflect that priority at all. A husband will claim that his wife and children are his priorities, but he will spend eighty hours a week at the office. An overweight person will admit that their health is very important to them, but they never exercise, and all they eat are unhealthy foods.

Taking care of your health is one of the wisest investments you will ever make. Some people say it's too expensive to eat healthy or they don't have time to exercise. I've said those same things myself. Of course, I would easily spend fifty bucks dining out, but wouldn't even think about paying that much money for a personal training session. I would never find fifteen minutes to exercise, but somehow I found two hours a night to watch TV. Get my drift?

It's all about priorities. In the past, my health was clearly not my priority. But it is now.

Even though my children, my marriage, being a good friend and sister are all priorities for me, my health must be my number one priority. I know now if I put my health in first place, then my loved ones will have a healthier, happier me for many years to come. Some of you worry that if you prioritize yourself first, then you'll be letting others down. The opposite is true. If you take time for yourself, it will help you to be a better mother, wife, and friend.

Mini-Challenge of the Day

Write down three things you value in order of importance. For example, maybe you value work, family, then your health. Be honest with yourself even if you have recently gotten your priorities mixed up. Review the list and circle the item that you consider your top priority. What priority are you giving your health? Is there an imbalance? How will you change your priorities to bring your life back in balance?

____

____

____

Tip of the Day

When making a quick and easy meal in a pan, such as scrambled eggs or seared tuna, use a cooking spray. Cooking sprays help you control how much oil you use and most of them are very low in calories. Some light versions have no calories. PAM cooking spray is one of my favorites. If you have to cook with oil, you can buy a refillable spray bottle and use that to spray your oil.

Meal	Record Your Food & Water Intake for the Day	Calories
1		
2		
3		
4		
5		
	Total Calories	

Fitness Plan

Cardio activity: ____________________ Time: ________ Miles: _____

Intensity level (circle one): L M H

Strength training (circle): Lower body Upper body Core

My Thoughts

____

____

____

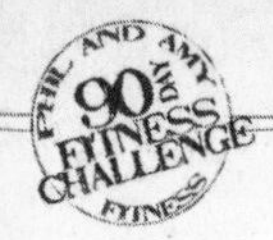

DAY 74—BEFORE THE DAWN

"Hope begins in the dark, the stubborn hope that if you just show up and try to do the right thing, the dawn will come. You wait and watch and work: you don't give up."

ANNE LAMOTT

A Note from Phil

Can you remember a time when you just didn't want to do something? I can. I had the hardest time this morning getting out for my daily run. I just didn't want to do it, but I knew I had to.

It was quite a battle. I had trouble getting out of the bed at 5 a.m. It was way too early. Then when I went outside, it was too cold. As I started running, all I could think about was how hard it was to breathe. Then my leg started to hurt. Everything was bothering me, and my body and mind were trying to get me to stop. But just like the Energizer bunny, I kept going and going and going.

As I neared the end of my run, the song "Yahweh" by U2 came on my iPod. It talks about how pain precedes the birth of a child. In other words, there is always struggle before a great achievement. When I heard that song, I felt the runner's high. It gave me the strength to push myself forward and finish my run. Endorphins and good feelings washed over me, and I felt a sense of accomplishment.

Why do we have to struggle to succeed? I don't know. But I do know that it's always darkest before the dawn. Each time you endure a deep struggle, it could very well mean that's the last step you have to climb before you get your breakthrough. I've heard that Thomas Edison tested some 3000 filaments before he came up with one that made the light bulb practical. I'm pretty sure by the 2999 test, he was wondering if he should just give up. But Edison didn't, and our whole world changed because of him.

Change the way you look at your specific struggle. Look at it as one step closer to your breakthrough. Keep moving toward your goals. The dawn will come if you don't quit!

Mini-Challenge of the Day

Name one thing you are struggling with today. Don't run from it. Work through it. Make yourself do what you don't want to do.

Tip of the Day

With obesity on the rise, type 2 diabetes is also on the rise. The American Diabetes Association says that twenty-one million people have diabetes and another fifty-four million people are in the prediabetic stage. Some complications of this common type of diabetes include heart disease, blindness, nerve damage, and kidney damage. If you are severely overweight, make sure you get tested. And stay motivated and healthy to avoid being at risk for this disease.

Meal	Record Your Food & Water Intake for the Day	Calories
1		
2		
3		
4		
5		
	Total Calories	

Fitness Plan

Cardio activity: ____________________ Time: ________ Miles: ______

Intensity level (circle one): L M H

Strength training (circle): Lower body Upper body Core

My Thoughts

____

____

____

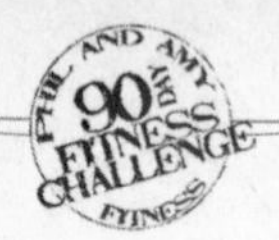

DAY 75—TRANSFORMATION

"I see it like a butterfly emerging from a cocoon. It'll take a while, but it'll spread its wings."
MICHAEL ROBINET

We adore Tabetha. Her excitement is contagious. Read what she has to say about her life transformation.

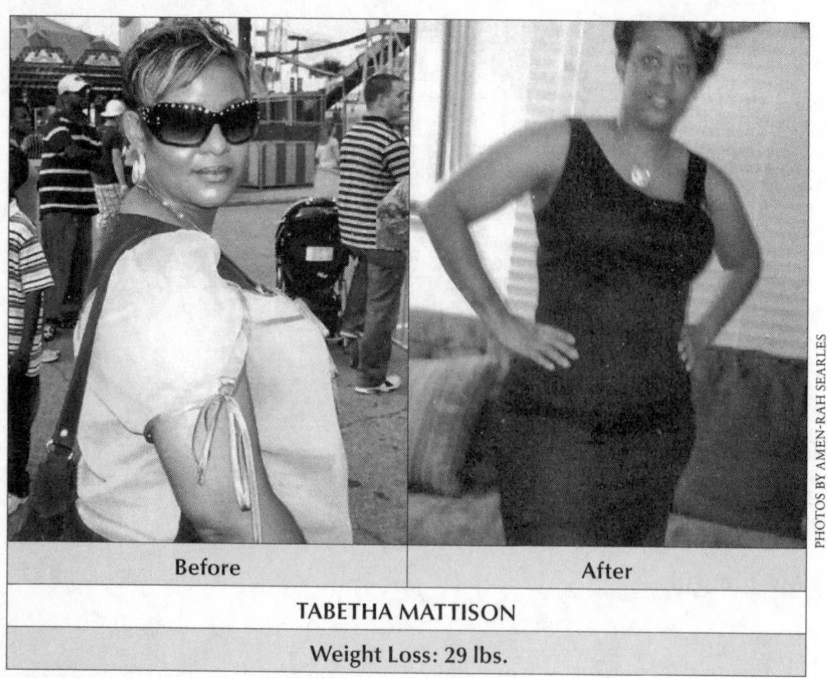

Before	After
TABETHA MATTISON	
Weight Loss: 29 lbs.	

PHOTOS BY AMEN-RAH SEARLES

"Thanks to the '90-Day Fitness Challenge,' I have a whole new way of life. The choices I make now are healthier, and I feel more in control of my life. I have broken from my cocoon and transformed into a butterfly. When anyone sees me today, they always see a butterfly on me somewhere—my shirt, my purse, or some other place—to represent the new me. I am so proud of myself and my success.

"When I started the 'Challenge,' I weighed 191 pounds. When it was over, I was down to a toned 162 pounds. I also went from a size 16-18 to a size 12-14 and can fit into some size 10s. That's amazing for me. I go to the gym three times a week, and I hired a trainer who keeps me motivated and challenged. I've kept the weight off now for a few months. My goal is to lose another 20 to 30 pounds, depending on how my body feels and adapts.

"I want to also stress the importance of having a weight-loss buddy. One of my best friends, Sandra Cortes, has been with me every step of the way. She is my motivator. I talk with her when I'm having a bad day, and she helps keep me on track. Another friend that I've known since college is also in this weight-loss program with me.

"I am so blessed to have the support not only from Phil and Amy through their daily emails but also from my good friends. I am a whole new person, and I hope that I can be an inspiration for others. If I can do it, you can do it."

Mini-Challenge of the Day

Send a thank-you email or postcard to a friend that has been helping and encouraging you along this process. They are a part of your success, and they would enjoy hearing how much you mean to them. Then do twenty pushups before you go to bed tonight.

Tip of the Day

Olive oil is one of the best oils to use for cooking and salads. Buy the ones that say "Virgin" or "Extra Virgin" on the label. These oils are the least processed and are healthier for your heart.

Meal	Record Your Food & Water Intake for the Day	Calories
1		
2		
3		
4		
5		
	Total Calories	

Fitness Plan

Cardio activity: ____________________ Time: ________ Miles: ______

Intensity level (circle one): L M H

Strength training (circle): Lower body Upper body Core

My Thoughts

____

____

____

Finishing Strong!
Putting It All Together for Life

Congratulations! You have almost made it to the end of the "Challenge." Let's check in and see how you're doing with everything you've learned so far. Let go of anything that's holding you back, lose the excuses, and learn to go with the ebb and flow of your journey...for the rest of your life.

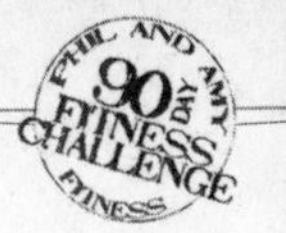

DAY 76—JUST CHECKING IN

"The great thing in the world is not so much where we stand, as in what direction we are moving."
Oliver Wendell Holmes

A Word from Amy

When you begin a project or task that's a big deal, it's a good idea to check in every now and then to see how you're doing. This is one way you can ensure that you meet your ultimate objective. This is especially important as it concerns weight loss. The end of the "90-Day Fitness Challenge" is closer than you think. You are already on Day 76, and today we're going to have a little check-up!

If you've been diligently following the "Challenge," then you should be excited to spend a few minutes to review what your efforts have accomplished. You've come a long way, and I applaud you for choosing to make a difference in your life. If you haven't stayed on track completely, this is a good time to get back with the program. We all fall down from time to time. The true test of our victory is if we stay down or choose to get back up.

I'm thankful that I have my husband as my accountability partner. We regularly keep each other in check and motivated to do the right things. If you haven't recruited someone to do the "Challenge" with you, then now is a good time to look for someone who can hold you accountable when you finish this program. You will need a support system of at least one person who can help you be honest about your daily eating and exercise habits. This can be a friend, a coworker, a family member, or even someone you meet online through our website.

Let's get started on your self-evaluation. Here is your pop quiz for the day. Write down the answers to the following questions. Be honest with yourself.

- What goal did you aim for at the beginning of the "Challenge"?
- How much progress have you made toward that goal?
- Are you using your food journal every day?
- Are you drinking enough water?
- Are you planning and cooking your meals on the weekend for the rest of the week?

- Are you eating five to six times per day?
- Are you consistently doing your cardio exercise and weight training?
- Are you getting the proper amount of sleep?

Give yourself a pat on the back for the areas where you are showing consistency. If there is any room for improvement, get back on track and focus on those areas the rest of the "Challenge." I know you can do it. You're almost there!

Mini-Challenge of the Day

Today, look at where you are and take stock. Pick three areas you answered above that you still need to work on. How are you going to get better in these areas? This is not the time to give up. It's the time to get even better!

____

____

____

Tip of the Day

Experiment with different kinds of green vegetables. Try bok choy, spaghetti squash, broccoli rabe, and savoy cabbage. Find recipes online to make a delicious meal out of these healthy and tasty ingredients.

Meal	Record Your Food & Water Intake for the Day	Calories
1		
2		
3		
4		
5		
	Total Calories	

Fitness Plan

Cardio activity: ______________________ Time: ________ Miles: ______

Intensity level (circle one): L M H

Strength training (circle): Lower body Upper body Core

My Thoughts

____

____

____

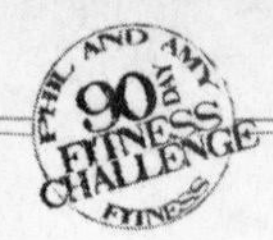

DAY 77—IT'S TIME TO PRUNE

"I am the true grapevine, and my Father is the gardener. He cuts off every branch of mine that doesn't produce fruit, and he prunes the branches that do bear fruit so they will produce even more."

JESUS (JOHN 15:1-2)

A Word from Amy

Every year before spring arrives, I prune my trees and bushes. It's hard work, but it's necessary so that my yard stays healthy and beautiful. Pruning clears away the dead branches and leaves and prepares the tree for new growth. Whenever I prune, I'm reminded of how applicable this is to our lives. At times we have to prune things from our lives in order to prepare us for new growth or a new level. In John 15:2, Jesus tells us that He prunes every branch that bears fruit so it can bear even more fruit. You are so close to the end of this "Challenge." Now is the perfect time to get rid of things that may hinder your race to the finish line.

Have you ever noticed that sometimes you have to give up one thing to get something else, something better, in return? We have to set aside savings to gain interest on our money. We have to make time for exercise so that our bodies are healthy. We have to plant a seed in the ground, and water and nourish that seed, so that we can grow a garden. We give up *x* and, in turn, we get *y*—something of value.

Is it time to prune? Are there things or even people in your life that are hurting you in some way? Some people around you might not support your health goals. I have a friend who began the weight-loss challenge and lost a lot of weight. Instead of being happy for her, her fiancé started to sabotage her efforts. He felt threatened and thought if she got in shape, she wouldn't love him anymore. If something similar has happened to you, you need to tell that person that, while you love and value them, your health is a big priority in your life. You might even have to disassociate with some friends temporarily so that you are strong enough to finish the course.

You might need to prune bad habits from your life. If you are anything like me, maybe you rely on food to comfort you in times of depression and stress. You will need to let go of these habits and replace them with better ones, such as eating healthy snacks, taking a long bath, or going to the gym.

Pruning is no easy task, and it can be painful. Always keep the goal in mind.

Pruning is necessary to make room for the new you. So let go of anything today that might be holding you back.

Mini-Challenge of the Day

Write down two areas in your life that need pruning. It can be anything that's preventing you from your growth. Make a commitment to prune that negative thing out of your life so you can finish strong.

____

____

____

Tip of the Day

Plan for life to throw you a curve ball as you continue on your weight-loss journey. You may have already experienced it. Just because the car needs tires, the kids need braces, or your great aunt died, it does not give you an excuse to get derailed from your food or exercise plan. Remember, emotion is not a part of this equation. Make a commitment to yourself that even though curve balls will come your way, you will stay the course.

Meal	Record Your Food & Water Intake for the Day	Calories
1		
2		
3		
4		
5		
	Total Calories	

Fitness Plan

Cardio activity: ________________ Time: _______ Miles: _____

Intensity level (circle one): L M H

Strength training (circle): Lower body Upper body Core

My Thoughts

____

____

____

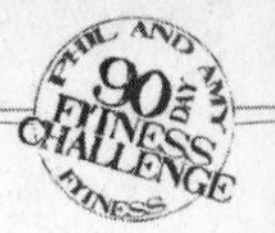

DAY 78—SEASONS OF LIFE

"Celebrate what you want to see more of!"
Thomas J. Peters

A Note from Phil

Yesterday was the most beautiful day. The birds were chirping, the sun was warm, the trees were blooming. The long winter was officially gone, and spring had arrived! Everyone was out riding their bikes, and children were laughing and playing in the park. The transition from cold, gray days to a warm and sunny one reminded me of what it's like going from a difficult season in life and coming out victorious on the other side.

The last few years for Amy and me have been a series of challenges and victories for our family. The challenges feel like the wintertime—cold, dark, with no end in sight. The victories feel just as euphoric and energizing as spring. We want it to last forever. Amy and I had our winter starting out on the show—experiencing grueling workouts, months of healthy eating, and many tears—and celebrated when our springtime arrived—standing on the scale at the grand finale and seeing how much weight we lost.

During this "Challenge" you've had to go through many seasons. I want you to think about the spring seasons. What have you conquered in the last few weeks that you are proud of? What has been a big aha moment for you? Where have you beat the odds and succeeded at something you never thought you could do?

Recently, I got an email from a couple participating in the "90-Day Fitness Challenge." They had written a list of things they were excited about since they had lost weight. They were grateful to easily fit into a restaurant booth. They now shop in the normal clothes department at the mall. They've saved money because they've taken the time to cook more at home. They no longer have to take their diabetes and blood pressure medications. In just weeks, this couple has shown some amazing results.

When they started their journey, it seemed like a long, hard road ahead. It was their winter season, and it's in this difficult season that we learn the most lessons.

But today let's reflect on the springtime victories. You can't have one without the other. It's time to enjoy the victories and benefits of your hard work. You've earned it!

Mini-Challenge of the Day

Take time today to reflect on your journey in the last few weeks. Write down five areas that you want to celebrate. Taking a moment to celebrate your accomplishments is just as important as putting in all the hard work to get there. I give you permission to go out today, find a healthy way to celebrate, and enjoy yourself.

____

____

____

Tip of the Day

Never eat only carbohydrates. For example, I always try to eat an egg with my cereal. If I ate cereal by itself, I would feel hungry again in about an hour. Adding just a bit of protein keeps my body more satisfied, and I won't feel like eating again until three or four hours later.

Meal	Record Your Food & Water Intake for the Day	Calories
1		
2		
3		
4		
5		
	Total Calories	

Fitness Plan

Cardio activity: ________________ Time: _______ Miles: _____

Intensity level (circle one): L M H

Strength training (circle): Lower body Upper body Core

My Thoughts

____

____

____

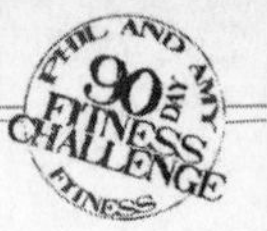

DAY 79—NO MORE EXCUSES

"Excuses are the nails used to build a house of failure."
DON WILDER AND BILL RECHIN

A Word from Amy

One of my college professors once told me that an excuse was "a skin of a reason stuffed with a lie." I never forgot that because I always had a good excuse why I couldn't get my homework in on time. Do you have the same problem? Are you an excuse maker? Too often we lie to ourselves about why we can't change our lives, why we can't work out, why we can't eat healthier.

When Phil and I got the call to be on the show, we had only a week's notice. We moved heaven and earth in those seven days so we could be on the show. We gave Phil's sister, who was watching our kids while we were away, power of attorney. We made sure our children were covered under our insurance policy. We sold a car in only five days to make sure we had enough money in the bank. We recruited help from our friends, neighbors, and our church to help us get ready and to help keep our house running while we were away. We packed clothes, wrote out schedules, and created lengthy to-do lists. We turned over all of our real estate listings to other agents in our office. It was a crazy time! I don't think Phil or I got more than three hours of sleep each night. We had the drive and motivation to get everything done in such a short time because we were not going to let this opportunity slip away.

We could have said that it was impossible, that we didn't have the money, and that the opportunity should just go to someone else. But we were serious and we meant business. We made miracles happen in that one week. It's amazing what can be accomplished when you stop the excuses and become determined to make things happen.

I know you want to change your life. You are already far into the "Challenge." Just make sure this "no-excuse" attitude will forever be a part of you. There is no reason you can't live the rest of your life healthy. Don't let excuses hold you back from living the best and longest life you can. Don't allow yourself to be fooled by the lies you tell yourself—that your results won't last or that you'll gain the weight back. Don't ever let excuses dictate your future.

Mini-Challenge of the Day

Face the truth. What is one area that you always have an excuse for? If you can't think of one, ask your friends. Now change those excuses into actions. If you say you can't get up in the morning to work out, you are lying to yourself. Prepare your clothes the night before, get to bed early, meet a friend at the gym, tell your spouse to kick you out of bed. Do whatever it takes to get you up the next morning.

Tip of the Day

Never, ever, ever skip breakfast. Eating breakfast is a key to successful weight loss. You will already be more successful if you eat just two eggs and a quarter cup of oatmeal for breakfast every day.

Meal	Record Your Food & Water Intake for the Day	Calories
1		
2		
3		
4		
5		
	Total Calories	

Fitness Plan

Cardio activity: ____________________ Time: ________ Miles: ______

Intensity level (circle one): L M H

Strength training (circle): Lower body Upper body Core

My Thoughts

____

____

____

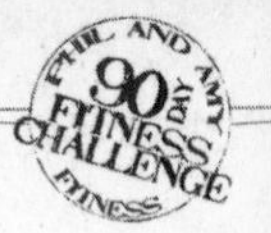

DAY 80—A CASE OF THE MONDAYS

"Don't you realize that in a race everyone runs, but only one person gets the prize? So run to win!"
PAUL (1 CORINTHIANS 9:24)

A Note from Phil

In the movie *Office Space*, the receptionist teases a coworker about having "a case of the Mondays." We all know what she's talking about. On Mondays, many people come into the office tired, bored, and not wanting to be there. You can probably hear someone say, "I can't wait until Friday." I'm sure we've all had a case of the Mondays, even in the middle of the week or on a day that's cloudy, rainy, and gloomy. All we want to do is hide under the covers until the day is brighter and there's something to look forward to.

Those days are just a part of life. I remember days on the weight-loss journey where discouragement would start to set in. It was usually a day when my charismatic personality wasn't blowing everyone away and no one seemed excited to see me. (I know, what a surprise, right?) Something just wasn't clicking or I was on a different wave length than everyone else. Many times it even made me want to quit my healthy lifestyle.

So what do you do when you have days like that? You do the right thing even if you don't feel like it. You don't quit. You don't change your course. You don't turn to food. You don't stay home instead of going to the gym. You keep on doing all the good things you've been doing. This is where your will, determination, and perseverance will make a difference.

Do you think the president of the United States feels like being president every day? I'm sure he wakes up every now and then and has a case of the Mondays. But he doesn't hide from the public. He faces his day just as he did the previous day. He does the right thing. He perseveres because he knows people depend on him.

As you come off this "Challenge," you'll need to keep motivating yourself when you have a bad day. Get the support of those who love you or who have traveled the same path. They will know what you're going through and will help you. Remember, this is not a temporary diet. This is a lifestyle change. Become good at dealing with these kinds of days because, every now and then, they will come.

Mini-Challenge of the Day

Are you having a case of the Mondays? However bad you feel right now, know that it won't last forever. You can change your attitude. Encourage yourself. Don't let it get the best of you. Your goal for today is to do all the good things you have been doing for yourself whether you feel like it or not. Eat well. Exercise. Drink water. Write in your food journal. The sun may not be shining in your day, but life has to go on. Keep making good choices.

Tip of the Day

Ever hear of exercise classes called Boot Camps? They're all the rage these days. Find out if your gym or local community center offers these classes. This is a great way to get in an hour of nonstop physical activity that will push your limits. You will do things you never thought you could do before and will see incredible results.

Meal	Record Your Food & Water Intake for the Day	Calories
1		
2		
3		
4		
5		
	Total Calories	

Fitness Plan

Cardio activity: ______________________ Time: ________ Miles: ______

Intensity level (circle one): L M H

Strength training (circle): Lower body Upper body Core

My Thoughts

____

____

____

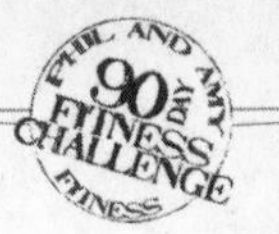

DAY 81—THANKFULNESS

"He is a wise man who does not grieve for the things which he has not, but rejoices for those which he has."
EPICTETUS

A Word from Amy

I am addicted to Facebook. There, I admitted it. It's one of my hobbies because I need constant stimulation. In just a few minutes, I can find out what all of my friends around the country are doing. It's like a big online reunion every day. On my "wall," I try to write down something that I'm thankful for. I've found that if I take the time to think about why I am grateful, my day already begins on a positive note.

The Bible tells us many times to be thankful. When we are thankful to God, we are praising Him for everything He has done in our lives. If our footsteps are always directed by God (Proverbs 16:9), then there is a reason for everything. That means we should be thankful for everything in our lives, not only what we believe to be the good things. It's all good!

I can find a way to be thankful for everything in my life. Even though bill collectors are calling, I am thankful that I have a house for my family to live in and cars to drive. Even though the dishwasher doesn't work, I am thankful that we have a beautiful set of dishes to eat our food on. I am thankful for my kids even when they leave fingerprints on the walls. It reminds me how fun our house is and how lucky I am to have a house full of happy kids. Even though we have some sibling rivalry, I am thankful for my brothers and sisters. They've made my life more interesting and passionate and filled with lots of love.

One of the most telling ways to be a positive person who succeeds is to maintain an attitude of gratitude. If we set our eyes on the positive, it expands our focus on good things. If you don't believe me, think about happy memories and how that makes you feel. I'm sure it makes you feel better and gives you a brighter outlook on the day. Now think about some bad memories. How does that make you feel? Depressed? Sad? Disappointed?

You are entering a whole new world with your weight loss. If you want to continue living a life that is healthy, don't forget to stay healthy on the inside. Be positive. Keep being thankful for all the blessings and opportunities you have.

Mini-Challenge of the Day

I suggested earlier that you keep a journal in your nightstand to write down what you are grateful for. Have you been doing that? If so, awesome! If not, I encourage you to get started. Right now, spend fifteen minutes writing down everything you are thankful for. You have a great life. Thank God for it.

Tip of the Day

Popcorn is a great snack, especially if you're watching a movie. Always make your own plain and unbuttered popcorn. Try the air popped kind, its less expensive and has less calories. One of my favorite things to put on popcorn is Crisco Butter Flavor Spray. It tastes better than some of the other sprays, and you get all the butter taste without all the calories.

Meal	Record Your Food & Water Intake for the Day	Calories
1		
2		
3		
4		
5		
	Total Calories	

Fitness Plan

Cardio activity: ____________________ Time: ________ Miles: ______

Intensity level (circle one): L M H

Strength training (circle): Lower body Upper body Core

My Thoughts

____

____

____

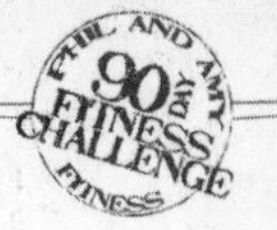

DAY 82—TEN THINGS TO KEEP DOING TO FINISH STRONG

"You don't make progress by standing on the sidelines, whimpering and complaining. You make progress by implementing ideas."

SHIRLEY HUFSTEDDLER

A Note from Phil

You are almost done! I know it's been an incredible journey so far, and I hope we hear from you about all the details. We all have stories to share on this "Challenge," and we'd love to hear yours.

With only nine days left to go, I want to remind you of the top ten things you need to do to finish strong and keep up your good, healthy habits. These are not just temporary changes you've implemented in your lifestyle; these are lasting changes, things that will keep you on the path to health for the rest of your life.

These reminders may seem redundant, but I cannot stress them enough. They are essential practices for you to follow regularly—as in all the time!

1. Buy a journal or a notebook and write down everything you eat. Be accountable to the page because the numbers don't lie.
2. Drink sixteen ounces of water when you get up in the morning. This will start your body moving and flush out your system.
3. Drink water all day. Make the decision that water will always be your drink of choice, and you love it.
4. Kick the salt. It's amazing how good food tastes once you get rid of the excess salt you put in it. Without it, you can really taste the natural flavorings, just as God intended us to without additives, preservatives, and extra stuff that's just not good for us.
5. Eat plenty of fruits and vegetables (at least five to six servings per day). Over 95 percent of Americans do not get enough fruits and vegetables. And no one ever got fat eating an apple.
6. Eat four to six small meals and snacks each day. No more starving yourself. Feed your body.
7. With each meal, combine protein, carbs, and a small dose of natural fat.

8. Eat like a king for breakfast. This should be your largest meal of the day.
9. Get up and move. Get at least thirty minutes of walking or movement most days.
10. Believe in yourself. You can do it! The power to change is within you.

Mini-Challenge of the Day

Think about specific habits you had difficulty with at the beginning of this "Challenge," but you eventually conquered. Maybe you hated water, and now you drink it every day and love it. Maybe you had self-esteem issues, and now your confidence level is at an all-time high. Write down these mountains you have climbed and let them encourage you to continue living a healthy life.

____

____

____

Tip of the Day

We spent ten bucks on a small food processer, and it's been one of the best additions to our kitchen. With this nifty gadget, we make our own salsa, hummus, and dips. Making these things from scratch lets you know exactly what's going into your food. And it takes no time at all.

Meal	Record Your Food & Water Intake for the Day	Calories
1		
2		
3		
4		
5		
	Total Calories	

Fitness Plan

Cardio activity: ____________________ Time: ________ Miles: ______

Intensity level (circle one): L M H

Strength training (circle): Lower body Upper body Core

My Thoughts

____

____

____

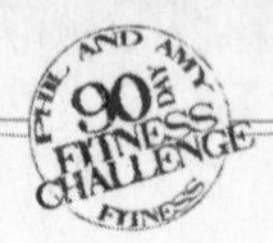

DAY 83—**ENERGY**

"The more you exercise, the more energetic you are."

Alexandra Lupu, Softpedia

Olivia dropped over 80 pounds the healthy way. She learned that gaining health has nothing to do with dieting; it's about making a permanent lifechange.

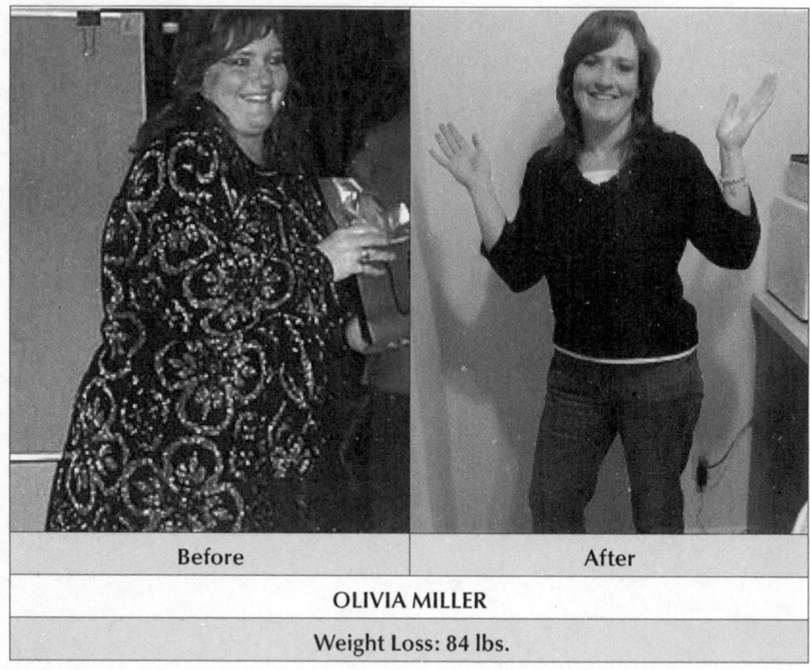

Before	After
OLIVIA MILLER	
Weight Loss: 84 lbs.	

"I went from a size 22 to a size 12 (from 246 pounds to 162 pounds) not by dieting but by changing my lifestyle. I am forty-three years old and have struggled with my weight for half my life. When I had my first son at twenty-one, I had gained 52 pounds. I lost only a little of that after giving birth. After my second son, I gained only 26 pounds. But throughout this time, I loved food and used it to comfort me. The weight kept packing on.

"I have been on just about every diet you can think of. I have lost some weight on a few of them, but I *always* gained it back quicker than I lost it. The reason I put the weight back on is that I pursued better health through dieting, not through a lifestyle change.

"I have been a fan of *The Biggest Loser* for the last four or five seasons. I watched it while I ate my ice cream or whatever I was craving that night. In December 2008, at my annual checkup with my doctor, I weighed 246 pounds. My parents are both diabetic, and I did not want to be diabetic too.

"After waking up to my poor health, I started 2009 with a commitment to a new lifestyle—eating healthier and exercising. When I joined Phil and Amy's 'Challenge,' I learned what worked for them and how their changes are long-term. They have taught me so much, and I have made so much progress in what I eat. I am fueling my body with better, lower calorie food and smaller portions but more often through the day.

"I am happy, healthy, and grateful to God, my family, my boss, and Phil and Amy—all of whom helped me get started on the right path to the person (and body) that I knew was hidden underneath."

Mini-Challenge of the Day

Go to the library or bookstore and visit the healthy lifestyle section. You'll find a lot of information, so don't get overwhelmed. Just pick up a few books you find interesting and discover a tip or two on a recipe or a new workout routine. It just might inspire you to see how others keep themselves healthy.

Tip of the Day

Plan your menus a week in advance and stick to the shopping list. You won't be tempted to buy on impulse, and you'll stick to your budget. Never forget that planning is one of the biggest keys to your success.

Meal	Record Your Food & Water Intake for the Day	Calories
1		
2		
3		
4		
5		
	Total Calories	

Fitness Plan

Cardio activity: ____________________ Time: ________ Miles: ______

Intensity level (circle one): L M H

Strength training (circle): Lower body Upper body Core

My Thoughts

____

____

____

Make a Difference in the Lives of Others: You Can Be an Inspiration

One of our greatest blessings in this "Challenge" is to give back to others. In what ways can you give and serve to help others? What kind of legacy will you leave for your family and the world? How will you make a difference?

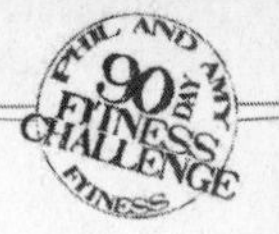

DAY 84—LEGACY

"We all can't leave a prestigious background or lots of money to our children, but we can leave them a legacy of love."
NAOMI RHODE

A Word from Amy

One of my father's hobbies was to explore graveyards and read the epitaphs on tombstones. It sounds pretty creepy, and in a way I guess it was. As a young girl, I would sometimes accompany him. I was always intrigued that a whole life could be reduced to a set of dates and a few words, such as *loving mother* or *caring brother.* Every time I would go on these excursions, on the way home I would think about what I wanted my legacy to be. What do I want people to remember about me? What do I want to leave behind? I realized the only way you leave a mark in this world is through how you make a difference in the lives of others—for the better or for the worse.

I want my life to count. I want to help people make their lives better. I want to share with others the blessings I've received. I want to teach my kids to become the best they can be. I want to leave an inheritance for my children. I want to be there for my friends when they need me. I want to be the best wife I can be to my husband. I want to inspire you to achieve your dreams.

I once read a survey that asked the participants to name one person who made a difference in their lives. Take a moment to think about how you would answer that question. Most of the folks who responded said it was a person close to them—either a friend, a parent, or a sibling. It's so easy to think that only rich and famous people make a difference—the Nobel Peace Prize winners or presidents or people whose names are in the headlines every day.

But that's not the case. We shouldn't think we matter less if the world doesn't know our name. What matters is how we make a difference in the lives of others. You have made incredible progress on your journey. You have made it through today with ups and with downs. You've learned great things. You've seen great changes. Now it's time to give back.

Make it your mission to help others around you, and you will leave a rich legacy. Take the gifts and talents you have and share them with others. Help someone else in their weight-loss journey. Share what you've learned with those on a similar path. You can make a big difference in the world, one person at a time.

Mini-Challenge of the Day

Think about the legacy you want to leave. Who do you want to help? Do you have a heart for helping your family, students, neighbors, homeless folks, foster children, orphans in other nations? What steps can you take to get started?

____

____

____

Tip of the Day

Eat on smaller plates. It will help you to eat less, and a full smaller plate is more appealing to the eye than a half-empty big plate. Some stores sell portion-control plates divided into sections as a way to retrain the user on how to eat.

Meal	Record Your Food & Water Intake for the Day	Calories
1		
2		
3		
4		
5		
	Total Calories	

Fitness Plan

Cardio activity: ________________ Time: _______ Miles: _____

Intensity level (circle one): L M H

Strength training (circle): Lower body Upper body Core

My Thoughts

____

____

____

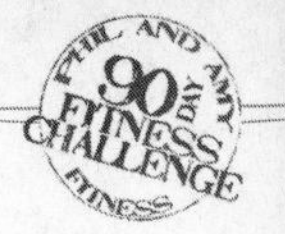

DAY 85—GIVING

"Balance, peace, and joy are the fruit of a successful life. It starts with recognizing your talents *and finding ways to serve others by using them."*
Thomas Kinkade

A Word from Amy

I am blessed to have a wonderful sister-in-law who has the heart of a giver. She sacrificed her time to watch our children while we were on the ranch. She took care of all our bills, our mail, and all household paperwork. She recruited other people in the neighborhood and church to help out so that everything was taken care of for us. When we got back, the house was in even better shape than when we left it.

The best part was that when I got home, my sister-in-law had almost an entire wardrobe ready for me in my new size. She had lost weight herself the previous few months and donated the clothes that no longer fit her to me. She also has a great sense of style, and some of the clothes she gave me I had admired and wished I fit into when I saw her wearing them. And now I could. What a gift!

I learned a lot from my sister-in-law about giving. I learned how to be selfless and give with a great attitude. I also saw that giving is not limited to donating money, as most of us think. There are many ways to give to others. You can donate your old clothes and furniture to charity or to your church. You can make a scrapbook of old photos for someone that will give them a lifetime of happiness. You can offer to babysit the children of the single working mother in your neighborhood. You can become a mentor for someone who is also on a weight-loss program. You can even give by just being the best person you can be. Just by doing that, you will be an inspiration to your friends and family.

As you reach the end of the "90-Day Fitness Challenge," it's all about doing for others. I'm sure along this journey someone has helped you in some way. Now it's time to pay it forward. Keep this attitude with you always, for it brings with it a cheerful heart and immediate personal satisfaction.

Maybe for you giving is hard to do right now. Just remember that the more you give, the more you make room to receive all the new blessings God has for you. Your metamorphosis is about transforming your life, so there will be a lot of opportunities to give away things that are no longer useful to you but are still useful to those around you. The best part about giving is joy. The more you give, the more joy you will have because you know you are making a difference.

Mini-Challenge of the Day

Think of one way you will give to someone who might be in need. For example, you might donate your older or larger-size clothing or something you have around the house. Be creative and keep it simple. Afterward, pay attention to how you feel. I'll bet that the act of giving leaves you with joy.

Tip of the Day

A lot of people tell me they need to lose weight *before* they join a gym so they can look good. I'm going to let you in on a secret—nobody cares. They're all too busy with their own health and looks. Don't postpone joining a gym because you're not thin enough. Do it today!

Meal	Record Your Food & Water Intake for the Day	Calories
1		
2		
3		
4		
5		
	Total Calories	

Fitness Plan

Cardio activity: ____________________ Time: ________ Miles: ______

Intensity level (circle one): L M H

Strength training (circle): Lower body Upper body Core

My Thoughts

____

____

____

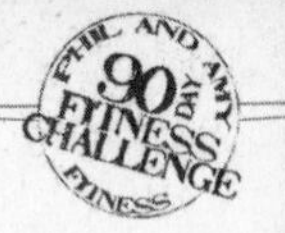

DAY 86—**SERVING**

"And whatever you do or say, do it as a representative of the Lord Jesus, giving thanks through him to God the Father."
Paul (Colossians 3:17)

A Word from Amy

I worked my way through college as a waitress. It was hard work spending long hours on my feet, carrying heavy trays, and keeping track of orders. Because the other waitresses and I relied on the customer for most of our income, we were all smiles when serving our tables. After all, the more friendly and helpful we were, the more tips we would make.

But out of earshot, many of the waitresses would complain and talk bad about customers, especially if they were rude or didn't leave a tip. Before I knew it, I was doing the same thing. I was saying some pretty mean things about those I served. I never felt good about myself when I did it, but it was a way that we all bonded back in the kitchen.

One day I decided that I would change my ways and serve all my customers as God would want me to. I felt too much of a fake talking bad about my customers behind their backs. I told myself that all they wanted was a good meal served promptly. Some of them might have had a hard day or a lot of stress in their lives.

Something strange and wonderful happened when I adopted my new attitude. When some of the customers gave me grief, I stopped taking it personally and remembered how I was there to serve them. I began to treat all my customers as if they were angels visiting my restaurant. When I stopped by their table, I brought a smile that came from my heart. I went above and beyond their requests and made sure they had a wonderful dining experience from beginning to end. I didn't care how big a tip they left me; I just made it my goal to serve my customers the best way I could, every day. While all the other waitresses were complaining, I was actually enjoying my job. And after only a few weeks, I was making the most money of all the waitresses in the restaurant.

Serving other people shouldn't be a chore. It should be a joy. We are here to serve and help other people. It's one of the ways you make a difference in the lives of others. You serve people every day, whether it's your coworkers, your spouse, your children, or your parents. Instead of complaining, serve in love the way God wants you to. You'll find that it will make your own life more fulfilling.

Mini-Challenge of the Day

What are some ways you are already serving others? Do you serve out of love or is it time for an attitude adjustment? As you go through today, be aware of all your interactions with others and how many times you are serving other people. You will be amazed at the many ways you serve people all day long. Before you go to bed, write down an opportunity you had to serve someone.

____

____

Tip of the Day

Surround yourself with friends who take care of their health and have a potluck dinner once a month. Have each person bring a home-cooked healthy meal and copies of the recipe. Not only is this a great way to catch up with friends, it's a way to try new foods and get new recipes.

Meal	Record Your Food & Water Intake for the Day	Calories
1		
2		
3		
4		
5		
	Total Calories	

Fitness Plan

Cardio activity: ____________________ Time: ________ Miles: ______

Intensity level (circle one): L M H

Strength training (circle): Lower body Upper body Core

My Thoughts

____

____

____

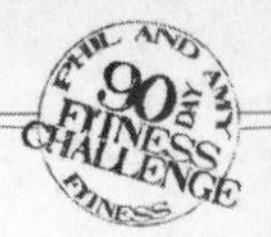

DAY 87—RECEIVING

"God has given us two hands: one to receive with and the other to give with."

BILLY GRAHAM

A Note from Amy

Imagine that in the next week, everyone you wanted to help in some way declined your offer. You offer to cook meals for a loved one who is ill, but they tell you they don't want to bother you. You offer to give your designer clothing to a family in need, but they politely refuse and suggest that you find another family to donate to. How would you feel? I imagine that after a while, you would stop wanting to give. After all, there is no joy in being rejected every time you offer to help.

I love to be independent. In the past, I didn't communicate what I wanted or needed because I thought I could handle everything myself. I discovered this year that there is more power when you allow people to use their God-given gifts to help you. Here's what I mean. I know very little about computers and websites, so recently I have asked for the advice of some acquaintances who are computer experts. Also, I have friends who are massage therapists, and I take them up on their offers of discount massages when I know my body needs one. Today I am more open to having others help me because it gives them joy to help (just as it gives me joy when I help others).

A woman who participated in the fitness challenge decided to start a personal assistant business. She does errands for busy people and takes care of their personal matters when they are out of town. She asked what my needs were and offered to do some errands for me for free. Her life changed so much after the fitness challenge that it gave her the courage to start her own business. Now she was ready to make a difference in other people's lives, and she started by donating her services to me.

Learn to accept that others can help you on your journey. The more you give and help others, the more you will find that people will help you. It will make you stronger when you allow yourself to put your ego aside and receive the gifts other people want to bless you with. So get ready to enjoy more of God's blessings!

Mini-Challenge of the Day

Remind yourself of these two responses: *Yes* and *Thank you*. The next time someone offers to help you, humbly accept their help with gratitude. It will bless your life, and you will also give the other person an opportunity to experience the joy of making a difference in your life.

Tip of the Day

Attend some sporting events in your area. You might find a sport you want to play yourself, you'll meet other like-minded people, and you'll be inspired to improve your own athletic skills after watching others.

Meal	Record Your Food & Water Intake for the Day	Calories
1		
2		
3		
4		
5		
	Total Calories	

Fitness Plan

Cardio activity: ____________________ Time: ________ Miles: ______

Intensity level (circle one): L M H

Strength training (circle): Lower body Upper body Core

My Thoughts

____

____

____

DAY 88—STEP IT UP: OUT GIVING GOD

"Remember that the happiest people are not those getting more, but those giving more."
H. Jackson Brown Jr.

A Word from Amy

Giving is such an important principle for making a difference; it teaches us to be involved in helping others and encourages us to always maintain a thankful heart and a willingness to contribute.

Have you ever heard the statement "You can't out give God"? I can tell you with certainty that it's true because I've experienced it. When we were living in Washington state, a guest speaker at our church talked about the importance of giving. I was so excited to contribute to the offering until I realized we didn't have any money. I knew there must be something I could give to God. Then I thought about the beautiful diamond ring my mother-in-law had given to me. I knew that was what I had to donate in the next offering. I did it without telling a soul.

What unfolded next sounds far-fetched, but I swear it's true. Within the next week, three different people had given me a car, a computer, and another diamond ring. I was so excited that I gave the car and the ring away to other people that I thought needed it more than I did. Within two weeks, someone else gave me a newer car, and checks totaling over a thousand dollars had come in the mail from various sources. It was crazy! I was so excited to keep giving—to help others and to thank God—and I learned I couldn't out give God. He is the ultimate gift giver.

Our primary intentions in giving should never be to get something in return. While it's the truth (Luke 6:38 NIV: "Give, and it will be given to you"), that's not why we give. We give because we are blessed and want to be a blessing to someone else.

The truth is that God loves giving so much that He rewards givers. Don't just take my word for it. Get out there and test this principle for yourself. Start with what feels comfortable to you. There are so many ways to give besides money. You can donate your car to a nonprofit cause or your time to a friend in need. The possibilities are endless.

Make giving a habit. Stretch yourself. And remember it's not a one-time deal. Do a little more this week than you did last week. Make a difference!

Mini-Challenge of the Day

Decide how you are going to out give God today. Give something that's out of your comfort zone, as I did with my diamond ring. Take a chance. With that positive thought in mind, pay attention in the next few weeks to the blessings you receive. Write down your experiences here.

____

____

____

Tip of the Day

For variety at the gym, use a mix of free weights and Nautilus equipment. Fixed-weight equipment is easy to use, especially if you're lifting heavy weights by yourself. Free weights are great for training your muscles on balance, coordination, and working on those smaller muscle groups. When you're at the gym, don't be shy if you're not sure how to use any of the weight machines. The trainers are there to help you.

Meal	Record Your Food & Water Intake for the Day	Calories
1		
2		
3		
4		
5		
	Total Calories	

Fitness Plan

Cardio activity: ________________ Time: _______ Miles: _____

Intensity level (circle one): L M H

Strength training (circle): Lower body Upper body Core

My Thoughts

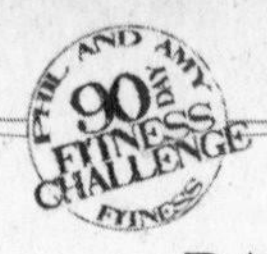

DAY 89—FOR EVERYTHING THERE IS A SEASON

"For everything there is a season,
a time for every activity under heaven."
Ecclesiastes 3:1

A Note from Phil

It's important for us to be aware of the different seasons in our lives because each season serves a different purpose. I had a long season of being overweight. I had a fear of scales, of doctors, and of gyms. I wasn't sure if I would even see my sons graduate from high school. I hoped I would see them get married and have their own kids, but I didn't know if I would because of my poor health.

Today I'm living in a new season. I have my health back and all those past fears have gone. I'm now able to help those who struggle with their weight because I can relate. I encourage and inspire others to become their best self because I know I was able to do it. I'm so fortunate to be able to make a difference in this way.

When you reflect on your past, remember that if you hadn't been challenged in some way and hadn't gone through difficult times, you probably would not have changed for the better. At the end of the "90-Day Fitness Challenge," you have accomplished most if not all of your goals. You have made significant strides in your health and lifestyle. You should be feeling great.

Guess what? You have officially entered a new season in your life. We want you to look around and see others who may be struggling in areas you have mastered. Think about someone who needs encouragement. Remember how difficult it was for you to walk even one mile at the beginning of this challenge? Look how far you've come! Now you can be a great encouragement to someone else at the beginning of their exercise program.

Remember the seasons of your own self-care. There is a time to help others and there is a time to help you. Always put your self-care first. If you take care of yourself, you'll have the energy and capacity to help others. If you spend too much time helping others, you'll drain yourself, and you might even let your good food and exercise habits start to slide. If you notice that to be true, take a break and put the focus back on yourself. There is a time and season for everything, and if you remember this, it will help to keep your life in balance.

You did it! You've ended the "Challenge." You've done an amazing job these last ninety days, and Amy and I are very proud of you. God bless you and keep it up. This is a lifestyle change, so keep going!

We want to hear about your experience. Email us at info@philandamyfitness.com and tell us about yourself. We would love to know how the "Challenge" changed your life for the better.

Mini-Challenge of the Day

Today, find someone who needs some help with weight loss and fitness. They might be interested in participating in the "90-Day Fitness Challenge," especially after they've seen your results. What is one thing you can do to inspire and encourage them to better health? Now go out and do it.

____

____

____

Tip of the Day

Have you heard of a bleacher run? It's a high-intensity workout that you should do at least once a week to boost your metabolism. You are now ready to try it out. Find a high school or college near you that has an athletic field with bleacher seats. For at least thirty minutes, run up and down the bleachers. This exercise will tone your legs significantly and give you a great cardio workout.

Meal	Record Your Food & Water Intake for the Day	Calories
1		
2		
3		
4		
5		
	Total Calories	

Fitness Plan

Cardio activity: ____________________ Time: ________ Miles: ______

Intensity level (circle one): L M H

Strength training (circle): Lower body Upper body Core

My Thoughts

____

____

____

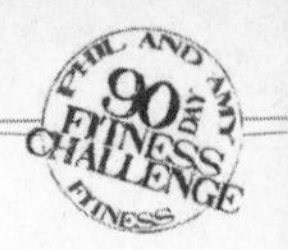

DAY 90—**WORK IT!**

"Movement is a medicine for creating change in a person's physical, emotional, and mental states."
CAROL WELCH

John and Rhonda Barth have lost over 160 pounds between them and remind us of how we started out on our health journey. We're so proud of their success.

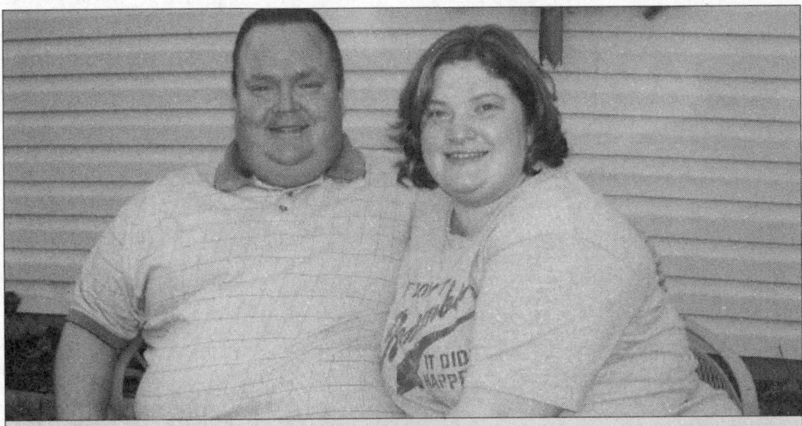

Before

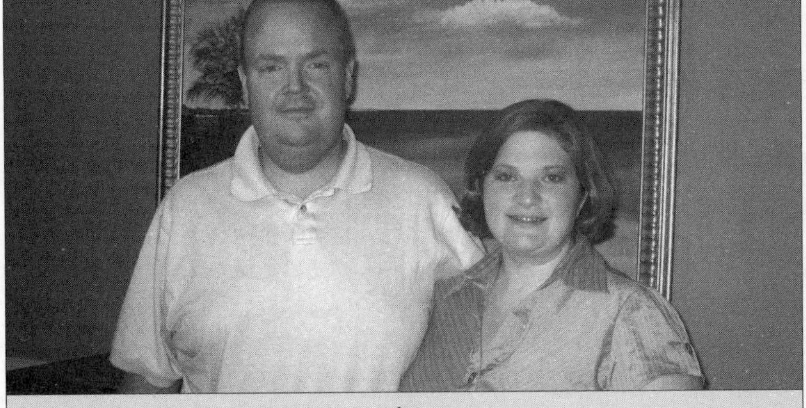

After

PHOTOS BY LINDA HERRING

JOHN AND RHONDA BARTH

Weight Loss: 95 lbs. (John), 66 lbs. (Rhonda)

(*John's Story*). "I've been heavy my entire life. I remember being astonished at my eighth-grade football physical when I weighed 172 pounds. It's no surprise that I ended up at 330 pounds by the time I was thirty-five with my diet of fast food, buffets, empty calorie drinks, and a sedentary lifestyle. I've lost weight in the past through myriad diets, but none has ever stuck. Phil and Amy's '90-Day Challenge' helped kick-start our journey toward healthiness.

"I began the 'Challenge' as a newly diagnosed diabetic and was informed that my blood pressure was high as well. By the end, I was on half-dose medication for both and have since become medication free. As my wife and I progressed through our journey, I realized that weight loss had become a secondary goal. We have taught ourselves how we need to eat, and we've finally embraced exercise and fitness as a necessary tool for improved fitness. Weight loss has become a by-product to our new lifestyle. We couldn't be happier.

"I wanted to set some new goals that weren't related to the scale, and I decided to take up running. I've since completed three 5K races, one 10K race, and will soon participate in a half-marathon. In the next several months, I hope to become a marathon runner as well. Not too bad for a guy who had been 100 pounds overweight for over half his life.

"Phil and Amy have provided the knowledge, guidance, and encouragement we've needed to get our lives back on track. They have proven that with desire, determination, motivation, and a bit of guidance, anything is possible."

(*Rhonda's Story*). "My husband and I have both experienced tremendous success so far and look forward to all the benefits of our new, healthier lifestyle. We've made exercise an integral part of our lives and strive to exercise every day. We have started walking outside, rather than on the treadmill, when the weather is decent, and we love the outdoors and spending time together.

"Recently I was out walking by myself, and the sun was hot and there was no breeze. I decided that I would walk one mile and then call it a day. For some reason, I kept walking after that first mile. When I had almost finished the second mile, I was even hotter and felt like stopping. But when I got to the intersection to turn toward our house, I kept walking straight. I didn't plan to walk that third mile, but I did it. By the end of that stretch, I was really hot and tired. But I had walked three miles.

"While I was walking, some part of my brain kept reminding me that what I was doing was uncomfortable and told me to quit. But some other part of my brain told my legs to keep moving. I accomplished my goal in spite of myself.

"In October, I walked a 5K, and I plan to run my first 5K soon."

Mini-Challenge of the Day

Today, jump rope for twenty minutes. Break it into intervals if you need to. This will get your heart rate up quickly. It's hard, but it's a great workout. That's why you see all the professional boxers jumping rope when they train.

Tip of the Day

Keep a calorie book in your car. It will help you choose your food wisely if you eat at a restaurant.

Meal	Record Your Food & Water Intake for the Day	Calories
1		
2		
3		
4		
5		
	Total Calories	

Fitness Plan

Cardio activity: ____________________ Time: ________ Miles: ______

Intensity level (circle one): L M H

Strength training (circle): Lower body Upper body Core

My Thoughts

____

____

____

Appendix A

Starting Point, Goals, and Final Outcome

My Starting Point on __________ (date)

Weight: _______

Blood pressure: _______

Body mass index (BMI): _______

Measurements:

_______ shoulders _______ hips

_______ chest _______ thighs

_______ waist

My Goals for this "Challenge" on __________ (date)

By _______ (date), I want to be _______ pounds.

By _______ (date), I want my blood pressure to read _______.

By _______ (date), I want my BMI to be _______.

By _______ (date), I want my measurements to be:

_______ shoulders _______ hips

_______ chest _______ thighs

_______ waist

The End Result of this "Challenge" on __________ (date):

Weight: _______

Blood pressure: _______

BMI: _______

Measurements:

_______ shoulders _______ hips

_______ chest _______ thighs

_______ waist

Appendix B

Shopping List

FRUITS and VEGETABLES

- ☐ Blueberries
- ☐ Strawberries
- ☐ Blackberries
- ☐ Raspberries
- ☐ Apples (all varieties)
- ☐ Lemon
- ☐ Lime
- ☐ Bananas
- ☐ Grapefruit
- ☐ Artichokes
- ☐ Spaghetti squash (not banana squash)
- ☐ Carrots
- ☐ Brussels sprouts
- ☐ Asparagus
- ☐ Broccoli
- ☐ Cauliflower
- ☐ Bell pepper (orange, red, green, yellow)
- ☐ Celery
- ☐ Cucumber
- ☐ Daikon
- ☐ Cilantro
- ☐ Mint
- ☐ Ginger root
- ☐ Endive
- ☐ Eggplant
- ☐ Garlic
- ☐ Jicama
- ☐ Lettuce (all varieties except iceberg)
- ☐ Spinach (regular or baby)
- ☐ Onions (white)
- ☐ Dried seaweed
- ☐ Sprouts
- ☐ Zucchini
- ☐ Tomato
- ☐ Cherry tomatoes
- ☐ Mushrooms
- ☐ Stir-fry vegetables (frozen)
- ☐ Green beans

RICE/BREADS/CARBS

- ☐ Wild long-grain rice
- ☐ Brown short-grain rice
- ☐ Whole-grain quinoa
- ☐ Brown-rice pasta
- ☐ Ezekiel bread
- ☐ Ezekiel buns
- ☐ Ezekiel tortillas
- ☐ Corn tortillas
- ☐ Low-carb whole-wheat tortillas
- ☐ 100 percent whole-wheat bread
- ☐ Steel-cut oatmeal
- ☐ Old-fashioned oatmeal
- ☐ Kashi GOLEAN waffles
- ☐ Kashi GOLEAN cereal
- ☐ Fiber One Original cereal

BEANS

- ☐ Chickpeas
- ☐ Edamame blanched-shelled soybeans (frozen)
- ☐ Fat-free, low-sodium black beans
- ☐ Dried lentils
- ☐ Great northern beans
- ☐ Red beans
- ☐ Black beans
- ☐ Low-sodium hummus

NUTS

- ☐ Dry-roasted almonds
- ☐ Raw walnuts
- ☐ Raw pecans
- ☐ Raw cashews
- ☐ Organic or all-natural peanut butter
- ☐ Hemp seed nuts
- ☐ Flax seeds or fiber

MEATS/FISH/PROTEINS

- ☐ Wild Alaskan salmon (not farm raised)
- ☐ Tilapia
- ☐ Tuna steaks (albacore and ahi)
- ☐ Tuna (canned, no salt)
- ☐ Alaskan black cod
- ☐ Catfish
- ☐ Alaskan halibut
- ☐ Chicken breast (organic, boneless, skinless, raw)
- ☐ No-salt sliced turkey breast
- ☐ Turkey (organic, ground turkey breast, and raw [previously frozen OK])
- ☐ Ground turkey
- ☐ Chicken (ground white meat)
- ☐ Turkey burgers
- ☐ Turkey sausage
- ☐ Uncured, no-nitrite turkey bacon
- ☐ Low-sodium roast beef
- ☐ Grass-fed beef (all kinds)

DAIRY

- ☐ AllWhites 100% Liquid Egg Whites
- ☐ Omega-3 whole eggs
- ☐ Non-fat sour cream
- ☐ Organic fat-free milk
- ☐ FAGE Total 2% greek yogurt
- ☐ Organic fat-free yogurt (FAGE Total 0%)
- ☐ Reduced-fat string cheese
- ☐ Laughing Cow Light Cheese Wedges
- ☐ Cottage cheese (low fat)
- ☐ Tzatzila Greek-strained yogurt dip

CONDIMENTS/DRESSINGS/OILS/SAUCES

- ☐ White balsamic vinegar
- ☐ Balsamic vinegar
- ☐ Rice wine vinegar
- ☐ No-carb BBQ sauce and ketchup
- ☐ No-sugar, low-sodium organic pasta sauce
- ☐ Galileo low-fat salad dressings (all flavors)

- ☐ Mustard (all varieties)
- ☐ Mayo (fat-free)
- ☐ Low-sodium, organic chicken broth
- ☐ Extra virgin olive oil
- ☐ Flaxseed oil
- ☐ I Can't Believe It's Not Butter Spray
- ☐ Cooking sprays
- ☐ Salsa

SEASONINGS and SPICES

- ☐ Allspice
- ☐ Basil
- ☐ Oregano
- ☐ Curry
- ☐ Turmeric
- ☐ Chili powder
- ☐ Crushed red pepper
- ☐ Dill
- ☐ Cinnamon
- ☐ Rosemary
- ☐ Pepper
- ☐ Cavender's Salt-Free Greek Seasoning
- ☐ Old Bay Seasoning
- ☐ Morton Salt Substitute
- ☐ Chef Paul Prudhomme's Magic Salt Free Seasoning
- ☐ Mrs. Dash Salt-Free Seasoning Blends

SWEETENERS

- ☐ Xylitol packets
- ☐ XyloSweet
- ☐ Stevia extract
- ☐ No-sugar, low glycemic jelly

COFFEE/TEAS

- ☐ Coffee (organic)
- ☐ Green tea (organic)
- ☐ Dandelion tea
- ☐ Lemon ginger tea (organic)
- ☐ Milk thistle tea (organic)
- ☐ Sparkling mineral water
- ☐ Unsweetened iced tea

NONDAIRY and JUICES

- ☐ Organic rice milk, almond milk, or soy milk
- ☐ Unsweetened cranberry juice (such as Knudsen Just Cranberry)

SNACKS

- ☐ Blue corn tortilla chips
- ☐ Snapea Crisps
- ☐ Wasa Whole Wheat Crispbread
- ☐ Streit's Matzos Unsalted
- ☐ Cuban crackers
- ☐ Whipped cream

Appendix C

Seven Daily Meal Plans

Day 1 Menu

Breakfast: Breakfast burrito. Scramble 3-4 egg whites, onions, mushrooms, some peppers, and low-fat Swiss or mozzarella cheese. Wrap it in a low-carb wheat wrap.

Midmorning Snack: Apple and 5-8 almonds

Lunch: The Amy salad. Mix fresh spinach, canned chicken (white meat), cherry tomatoes, cucumbers, raisins, and a sprinkle of walnuts. Toss with oil and vinegar, salsa, or mustard.

Afternoon Snack: One string cheese and a plum or other seasonal fruit

Dinner: Grilled salmon, asparagus, and half a sweet potato

Day 2 Menu

Breakfast: Ground turkey scramble. Take 1 cup of cooked ground turkey, scramble with 3 egg whites, spinach, red peppers, garlic powder, and salt substitute. Serve with a slice of whole wheat or Ezekiel bread.

Midmorning Snack: One tangerine and ¼ cup of walnuts

Lunch: Chicken pita. Stuff a whole wheat pita with 4-6 ounces of cooked chicken tenderloins, spinach, artichokes, bell peppers, sprouts, onion, and tomato. Use spicy mustard or hummus for dressing. Eat with 16 organic, blue corn tortilla chips.

Afternoon Snack: Greek yogurt with fresh berries and Xylitol or Stevia to taste

Dinner: Cooked tilapia with ½ cup brown rice, salsa if desired, and steamed broccoli

Day 3 Menu

Breakfast: Cook 4 egg whites any way you choose, 2 slices of cooked turkey bacon (no nitrates), 1 slice of Ezekiel toast, ½ cup low fat cottage cheese

Midmorning Snack: Fuji apple and 5-10 almonds

Lunch: Peanut butter and jelly sandwich made with 1½ tablespoons of natural peanut butter and 1 tablespoon of all-fruit jam on whole wheat or Ezekiel bread. Side of raw carrots.

Afternoon Snack: Cuban crackers with 2 tablespoons of hummus

Dinner: Turkey burgers made with 93 percent lean ground turkey and 100-calorie whole wheat buns. Garnish with spinach, tomato, sprouts and Laughing Cow low-calorie Swiss cheese. Eat with a side of sweet potato fries. (Slice sweet potatoes, spray with nonstick cooking spray, brush lightly with honey and a little cayenne pepper, and bake them in oven until soft.)

Day 4 Menu

Breakfast: One-half cup Fiber One (the original) cereal plus ½ cup Kashi GOLEAN cereal with 1 cup skim/soy or 60 calorie almond milk. Cook 2 egg whites any style.

Midmorning Snack: A boiled egg and an apple

Lunch: Turkey sandwich made with low-sodium turkey slices, bean sprouts, tomatoes, and spinach with spicy, brown mustard on sprouted, multi-grain bread. Side of mixed fresh fruit.

Afternoon Snack: One rice cake with 1 tablespoon peanut butter and half a banana

Dinner: Baked chicken (without skin) with sodium-free seasonings. Serve with 2 cups steamed vegetables, ½ cup brown rice with salsa or hummus if desired, and strawberries for dessert.

Day 5 Menu

Breakfast: Two eggs cooked any style and ½ cup old-fashioned oatmeal with cinnamon or Stevia, if desired

Midmorning Snack: Broccoli and carrots with olive hummus

Lunch: Tuna sandwich and an apple or other piece of fruit. Mix canned tuna, chickpeas, 1 tablespoon of olive oil, mustard and dill, and spread on whole wheat or Ezekiel bread with tomato and lettuce.

Afternoon Snack: Wasa crackers with Laughing Cow cheese or peanut butter

Dinner: Chicken burgers. Make a chicken patty with lean, ground chicken, cooked kidney, black, or navy beans, 1 egg, green peppers and onions, salt substitute, garlic or other spices. Eat on 100-calorie whole wheat buns with Laughing Cow cheese and mustard. Side of ½ cup brown rice with spices of your choosing and 1 cup of steamed vegetables.

Day 6 Menu

Breakfast: Ezekiel French toast. Dip 2 slices of Ezekiel bread in egg whites, cook on nonstick skillet, and top with fresh berries or jam and agave nectar for syrup.

Midmorning Snack: One tablespoon guacamole and organic blue corn tortilla chips

Lunch: Cooked chicken tenderloins with ½ cup of brown rice with salsa and steamed broccoli

Afternoon Snack: Nonfat frozen yogurt with almonds or peanut butter

Dinner: Salmon with light butter, steamed vegetables, and a sweet potato

Day 7 Menu

Breakfast: Organic buckwheat pancakes with strawberries and agave nectar, and a side of turkey bacon (no nitrates)

Midmorning Snack: Orange and 2 rice cakes

Lunch: Bean soup. Mix cooked kidney, black bean, or navy beans with tomatoes, red peppers, and onions, and simmer in low-sodium chicken broth.

Afternoon Snack: One cup of cottage cheese and piece of fruit

Dinner: Whole-wheat spaghetti made with homemade spaghetti sauce (chopped canned tomatoes, tomato paste, oregano, sliced mushrooms, olive oil, black pepper, and salt substitute). Side green salad with vegetables of your choosing.

Appendix D

Recipes*

Southern Comfort Lime Chicken

(1 serving = 1 chicken breast)

Ingredients:

1 cup fresh lime juice
½ cup fresh orange juice
1 jalapeno, seeded and minced
2 teaspoons kosher salt
1 teaspoon fresh ground pepper
1 tablespoon minced garlic
1 tablespoon chili powder
½ teaspoon cumin
6 boneless chicken breasts

Directions: Mix all the ingredients above except the chicken. Marinate chicken in this dressing 8–24 hours before grilling, basting twice.

Garlic Ranch Dressing

(1 serving = 2 tablespoons)

Ingredients:

½ cup light mayonnaise
¼ cup grated light parmesan cheese
¼ cup nonfat buttermilk
1½ tablespoons minced garlic
1 teaspoon minced flat leaf parsley
To taste ½–1 cup apple cider vinegar

Directions: In a bowl, whisk together all ingredients except vinegar. Add vinegar to taste and consistency desired. Chill for 2 hours.

---

* All recipes in this appendix have been contributed by our friend Tim Polin unless otherwise indicated.

Salmon Fillets

(1 serving = 1 fillet)

Ingredients:

4 salmon fillets

1 cup orange juice

2 tablespoons low-sodium soy sauce

1 bunch of fresh dill

cedar paper

fresh ground pepper

Directions: Marinate salmon in orange juice, soy sauce, and 1 tablespoon chopped dill for 2 hours. Before cooking, add pepper and 1 sprig of dill to each fillet. Grill to desired temperature skin-side down on cedar paper.

Graham Cracker Sammy

Ingredients:

Low-fat graham crackers

Fat-free whipped topping

Directions: Line a 9x12 baking dish with 1 layer of crackers broken into smaller sections. Spread whipped topping over the crackers. Add another layer of crackers and spread another layer of topping. Repeat as necessary. Place in freezer for 2 hours.

Tim's Fantastic Fajitas

Ingredients:

1 package fajita seasoning mix

2 large boneless skinless chicken breasts

1 large onion, sliced into strips

2 bell peppers, sliced

1 teaspoon olive oil

whole-wheat flour or low-carb tortillas

Directions: Place chicken in freezer for 20-30 minutes or until just starting to freeze. Remove and cut into thin strips. Heat oil and cook until chicken is brown. Set aside. Sauté onion and pepper until soft. In a small bowl, mix fajita seasoning and water as indicated on package. Add mix to vegetables, add chicken, and simmer to reduce liquid. Place tortillas in wet paper towels in microwave for 30 seconds or until hot. Serve together.

*Black Bean Hummus**

Ingredients:
1 can black beans
½ teaspoon minced garlic
1 teaspoon kosher salt
⅛ teaspoon cayenne pepper
3 tablespoons lime juice
¼ cup tahini paste
¼ cup olive oil
¼ cup water
1 teaspoon cumin
1 teaspoon coriander

Directions: Mix all ingredients in a food processor until smooth. Eat with whole-wheat bread or organic chips.

* Recipe provided by www.scratchmeals.com

Appendix E

Workout Plans

We have created a three-tier plan for you to follow on this "Challenge." Each plan contains cardio options and weight-training exercises and increases in intensity every thirty days.

Cardio

Cardiovascular activity, which basically burns fat, needs to be the backbone of your workout plan. Be creative. You don't have to stick to our options. You can dance, play in the backyard with your children, or play a sport. We suggest doing 30–60 minutes of cardio 5–6 times a week (each plan targets a specific duration for that particular time period). Don't feel as though you have to do one exercise for your entire workout. For example, you can do one activity for 20 minutes and another for 20 minutes. The most important thing is to keep your heart rate up during this time.

Before you start any cardio exercise, it's important to stretch and warm-up for 5–10 minutes. Finish a workout the same way. You want to avoid injury at all costs. One more thing: if you are going to do cardio on a day you plan on strength training, I recommend lifting weights first, then cardio.

Resistance Training

Resistance training is important to build muscle and to make you look tight and toned. If all you did was cardio, you would just be a smaller and saggy version of your same shape. Resistance training will transform your body shape, and you will be stronger and feel more confident.

The three plans we outline for you are performed with your own body weight in addition to basic equipment you can buy at your local sporting goods store. These include: workout bands (at least three bands with different resistance levels), dumbbells (pair of 3-lb., 5-lb., 8-lb., 10-lb., and 15-lb.). You should increase weight up or down accordingly. Remember the key is resistance. We want you to be able to work out in the privacy of your own home at first, if that's what you are most comfortable with. If you decide to join a gym, you will have more options using weight training equipment; that's up to you. The best part about the equipment used in our workout plans is that most of it comes with instructions or free videos on how to use it.

When using dumbbells, you may need to increase or lower the weight we suggest depending on your level of strength. You know you are using a good weight if by the last two reps, you are exerting a lot of effort, even struggling, to complete them. You'll know if the weight we suggest is too light if you are able to complete the number of suggested reps without much effort. If that's the case, increase your weight.

Our workout plan is focused on lower body (gluts, quads, hamstrings, calves), upper body (shoulders, arms, chest, and back), and abdominals. The whole set of these exercises can be performed in one session and should take 45 minutes to 60 minutes. Throughout the "Challenge," you will want to do resistance training three times per week on nonconsecutive days (your body needs to recover).

All exercises will be performed for two to three sets. One set is 10–15 repetitions of the exercise. You will need about 30 seconds to one minute to recover between each set. For example, you will do Set 1 of 10–15 reps. Rest one minute. Then do the second set for 10–15 reps. And so on.

You can begin with either lower body or upper body, but always end each resistance training session with the abdominal exercises. Amy and I normally exercise the largest muscles first and the smallest muscles last. For example, for upper body, you will exercise the back muscles before the triceps.

Plan 1 for Days 1–30

Cardio

This plan should be fun and easy. Work out at least four times per week at a minimum of 30 minutes. If you can work out for more, great! Just don't burn yourself out. You don't even have to join a gym at this point. The easiest kind of cardio to do right now is to walk. Put on your sneakers and walk around your block for 30 minutes. It's simple and effective. Here are some walking ideas and other forms of cardio you can choose to do for the first 30 days of the "Challenge":

- Walk on a treadmill.
- Walk around your neighborhood.

- Walk on a hiking trail in a local park.
- Walk around a local high-school track.
- Take your dog for a brisk walk.
- If you have a baby, take the baby out for a walk with the stroller.
- Walk up and down some hills for variety.
- Dance inside your house with high-energy music at your own pace.
- Rake leaves.
- Do some housework, such as vacuuming or mopping the floors.
- Do a physical activity with your children and keep your heart rate up.
- Have a bike at home? Take it for a ride around the neighborhood.
- Rent a cardio DVD from the library and exercise to it in your living room at your own pace.
- Swim or do aqua aerobics at your community swimming pool.

Resistance Training

Upper-body exercises

1) *Pushups* (works entire upper body)—2 sets of 10 reps

Pushups use most of the muscles in your upper body. They are one of the best exercises to tone up your upper body without using any equipment. Start with wall or knee pushups.

Wall: Stand up, facing the wall. Arms should be shoulder-length apart. Lower your chest toward wall. Try to keep back straight as you push back up.

Knee pushups: Lie on your stomach, then push up with your arms, keeping your back straight. Your arms should be shoulder-length apart and your knees on the floor. Lower your chest back toward the floor, again keeping your back straight.

2) *Bent-over row* (strengthens back)—2 sets of 10 reps with 10-lb. dumbbells.

Place your right knee and hand on a bench with your back straight and parallel to the floor. Hold a dumbbell in your left hand, allowing your arm to hang toward the floor. Keeping your back flat, lift the weight toward your hip until your elbow bends past 90 degrees and your upper arm is in line with your back. Hold, then slowly return the weight to the start position. Repeat with same arm, and then switch arms.

3) *Three-way raise* (strengthens chest)—2 sets of 10 reps

Start by placing the resistance band on the floor. Stand on the band in the middle with your feet shoulder width apart. Grab the handles. Then raise your arms straight out from your sides until they are parallel to the floor. Lower to starting position, then raise your arms straight in front of you with your arms together. Lower to starting position. Then hold the handles in front of your body with your hands together, knuckles facing forward, and raise the bands to your chest. Your elbows should be pointed out and parallel to the floor. Do each of these exercises 10 times.

4) *Chest flys* (strengthens chest)—3 sets of 12 reps with 10-lb. dumbbells

Lie down on a bench. Hold the dumbbells at arm's length above you with palms facing each other. Now lower the dumbbells as far as possible on the sides as you push your chest out. Return the weights to the starting position above you.

5) *Shoulder press*—3 sets of 10 reps

Stand on the resistance band with your feet shoulder width apart. Grasp the handles with an overhand grip and raise your hands to shoulder level, palms facing forward. Press resistance bands upward. Lower and repeat. Keep back straight as possible.

5) *Bicep curls* (strengthens biceps)—3 sets of 10 reps

Stand on the resistance band with your feet shoulder width apart. Grasp one handle in each hand, palms facing inward. Keep back straight and use your arms to stretch the bands toward your shoulders, tensing your biceps at the top. Slowly lower your hands to the starting position. Do not let the band collapse as you go down, but keep tension on it.

6) *Chair dips* (strengthens triceps)—3 sets of 10 reps

Sit on edge of chair or bench, legs extended in front of you, hands at your side on the chair. Heels and feet should be supporting you. Drop down lowering your hips to toward the floor. Push yourself back up by straightening your arms.

Lower-body exercises. Squats and lunges are some of the best exercises to tone up your leg muscles, so our plans are focused around on them. These exercises work out your entire leg as well as your gluts.

1) *Body-weighted squats*—3 sets of 10–15 reps

Begin with feet shoulder width apart and arms in front of you. Keeping back straight, squat down until your thighs are parallel to floor. Press up from heels and return to starting position. This exercise, if done correctly, can tighten your thighs, hips, and bottom. Do squats as deep as your body allows.

2) *Standard lunge*—2 sets of 10 reps

Begin with both legs together. Move one leg forward about two feet and lower your front thigh until it is almost parallel with the floor. Concentrate on keeping your back straight and going straight down, not falling forward. This is a common mistake. You want to keep good form. Be careful not to hyperextend your knee. I always make sure my knee does not go over my toe. Next, push yourself up and continue lunging down until reps are done. Switch to other leg.

3) *Walking lunge*—2 sets of 10 steps for each leg

The walking lunge is the same as a standard lunge except you move yourself forward as you do each one, as if you were walking. (See instructions for the *standard lunge*.) As you push up off the toes of your back foot, push your body forward to land your back foot in front, and then do another lunge. Keep moving forward with each lunge that you do.

4) *Step ups*—3 sets of 10 steps for each leg

You'll need a step, stairway, box, platform, or low bench for this one. Starting with both feet on the floor, step up with one leg, then with the other. Return to your starting position one leg at a time. Repeat this process.

5) *Calf raises*—2 sets of 15 reps for each leg

Stand with feet about six inches apart on the edge of a step. Lower your heels as far as possible in a good stretch. Keep your knees straight but not locked. Then rise up onto the balls of your feet and squeeze your calf muscles. This is one calf raise. Repeat.

Abdominal exercises. It's important to work your abs at least three times a week. They are considered core muscles. Strong abdominal muscles support your back muscles and help prevent injury. Here are a few exercises you can do.

1) *Sit ups with inflatable ball*—30 reps

Lie back on the inflatable ball. Your feet are planted flat on the floor. Your upper back is lying toward the back of the ball. With both hands behind your head, sit up doing a crunch. Lie back down. This is one rep.

2) *Leg lifts*—20 reps

Lie on the floor. Keep your hands either under your buttocks or next to you. Squeezing your abdominal muscles, raise both legs at the same time until your feet are 6 inches off the floor. Hold for 5–10 seconds. Lower. When you raise your legs, they should be together, not apart.

3) *Bicycles*—2 sets of 15

Lie on the floor. Place hands behind your head. Raise your right leg slightly as you bend your left leg up, bringing it toward your chest. Tense your abs and do a crunch by bringing your right elbow toward your bent left knee. Now alternate your leg position as if you were riding a bike, bringing the opposite leg toward your chest and bringing your left elbow toward your bent right knee.

4) Abdominal crunch (basic)—2 sets of 10

Lie on your back, bend your knees, and place your hands on the side of your head. Contract your abs and flatten your lower back against the floor. Slowly lift your shoulder blades one or two inches off the floor. Hold for a few seconds. Slowly lower while keeping your abs contracted.

5) *Vertical leg crunch*—2 sets of 10 reps

Lie on the floor, face up. Extend your legs straight up with your knees crossed. Crunch your abs by lifting your shoulder blades off the floor as if reaching your chest toward your feet; keep your eyes on the ceiling. Keep your legs always extended and in a fixed position. Lower and repeat.

Plan 2 for Days 31–60

Cardio

This second tier of the workout plan is about trying new exercises for variety and increasing your intensity. Aim to do 30–45 minutes of cardio, 5–6 times per week. You can still do Plan 1 exercises, just increase the time and intensity. For example, if you have been walking, instead of doing that for 45 minutes, alternate walking with a minute of light jogging several times within that session. Below are more cardio examples. Some of these machines and classes you will find at your local gym if you decide to join one at this point in the "Challenge."

- walking mixed with light jogging
- light jump roping

- cardio equipment, including the treadmill, elliptical machine, stationary bike, rowing machine
- classes at your local gym that focus on cardio at a beginner or intermediate level, including step classes or aerobic classes
- fitness shows that air on TV

Resistance Training

Upper-body exercises

1) *Regular pushup*—2 sets of 10 reps

Lie down facing the floor; arms should be shoulder length apart. Try to keep your back straight as you push up until your arms are fully extended, but avoid locking your elbows. Then slowly lower your chest toward the floor.

2) *Bent-over row*—2 sets of 12 reps with a higher weight dumbbell (see previous description of this exercise)

3) *Intermediate three-way raises*—3 sets of 12 reps with a stronger resistance band (see previous description of this exercise)

4) *Chest flys*—3 sets of 15 reps with a higher weight dumbbell (see previous description of this exercise)

5) *Single-arm bicep curl with resistance bands*—3 sets of 10 reps

Stand on the resistance band with your feet shoulder width apart. Hold both handles in your right hand with your palm facing outward. Keep back straight and use your arm to pull the band upward toward your right shoulder, tensing your bicep at the top. Slowly lower the band to the starting position. Do not let the band collapse as you go down, but keep tension on it. Repeat with the left arm.

6) *Shoulder press*—3 sets of 10 reps with 10-lb. dumbbells

Grasp the dumbbells with an overhand grip and hold them at shoulder level, palms facing forward. Press dumbbell upward. Lower and repeat. Keep back straight as possible.

7) *Bicep curls*—2 sets of 10 reps with 15-lb. dumbbells

With your feet shoulder width apart, hold one dumbbell in each hand, palms toward your sides. Keeping your back straight, bend your elbows and use your biceps to pull the weights toward your shoulders, tensing your biceps at the top. Slowly lower the dumbbell to the starting position. Do not let the weight collapse as you go down, but keep tension on it.

8) *Chair dips*—3 sets of 15 or more reps (see previous description of this exercise)

Lower-body exercises (see previous descriptions of these exercises)

1) *Body-weighted squats*—3 sets of 10–15 reps

2) *Standard lunge*—3 sets of 10 reps and add 5-lb. dumbbell in each hand

3) *Walking lunge*—2 sets of 15 steps for each leg and add 5-lb. dumbbell in each hand

4) *Step ups*—3 sets with 15 reps and add 5-lb. dumbbell in each hand

5) *Calf raises*—3 sets with 15 reps for each leg and add 5-lb. dumbbell in each hand

Abdominal exercises (see previous descriptions of these exercises)

1) *Sit ups with inflatable ball*—50 reps

2) *Leg lifts*—40 reps

3) *Bicycles*—3 sets of 15

4) *Abdominal crunch*—2 sets of 15 reps

5) *Vertical leg crunch*—2 sets of 15 reps

Plan 3 for Days 61–90

Cardio

The third tier of the workout plan is about pushing yourself every time you work out. By now you have built up some endurance and have gotten a lot stronger since you started. Continue to do cardio 5–6 days per week and increase your workout times to 45–60 minutes. You can still use the same options in Plan 2, just increase the intensity. Don't be afraid to try new machines and new classes at the gym. Here are some options:

- walking mixed with longer intervals of jogging

- jogging
- rollerblading
- mountain biking
- sports such as tennis, soccer, basketball
- running bleachers at a local high school
- StairMaster or step machines
- classes at the gym, including spin, kickboxing, and higher-intensity aerobics

Resistance Training

Upper-body exercises (see previous descriptions of these exercises)

1) *The pushup with variations*—3 sets of 10 reps

Do a regular pushup with variations. For example, spread your arms wider apart or move them closer together before you lower your chest. You can also put your legs on a bench for elevation and then lower your chest. This creates additional resistance.

2) *Bent-over row*—3 sets of 12 reps with a higher-weight dumbbell

3) *Chest press*—3 sets of 12 reps with 15-lb. (or more) dumbbell

4) *Chest flys*—3 sets of 12 reps with 10-lb. (or more) dumbbell

5) *Shoulder press*—3 sets of 12 reps with 10-lb. (or more) dumbbell

6) *Bicep curls*—3 sets of 12 reps with 15-lb. (or more) dumbbell

7) *Chair dips*—3 sets of 20 reps

Lower-body exercises (see previous descriptions for most of these exercises)

1) *Body-weighted squats*—4 sets of 15-20 reps

2) *Jump lunge*—3 sets of 12 reps

Step 1: Stand up straight with your feet shoulder width apart, but with one about a foot and a half in front of the other. Your back leg should be directly under your body, and your forward leg bent at ninety-degree angles at the knee and hip. Hold your arms straight out in front of you. Keep your torso straight throughout the exercise.

Step 2: Jump off the floor slightly and quickly switch the position of your feet in midair.

Step 3: Land in the mirror-image of your original position—your forward leg bent at the knee and hip and your back leg directly underneath your body. Bend your knees to absorb the impact, but keep your feet and knees facing straight forward.

Step 4: Jump back off the floor, switching your feet to your original position.

3) *Walking lunge*—2 sets with 20 steps and add 8-lb. dumbbell in each hand

4) *Step ups*—3 sets of 20 steps and add 8-lb. dumbbell in each hand

5) *Calf raises*—3 sets with 20 steps and add 10-lb. dumbbell in each hand

Step 1: Assume your starting position on the floor and hold a 10-lb. weight in each hand. Your arms should hang by your sides in a natural relaxed position throughout the movement. Stand with your heels at hip-width position.

Step 2: Raise your heels off the floor until you are standing on your tiptoes and hold this fully extended position for a moment. Lower your heels until they are just about to touch the floor and immediately begin your second repetition.

Step 3: Perform about 15 reps. Calf muscles, because they are well designed for frequent use, benefit more from reps than any part of the body other than the abdominals.

Step 4: Do calf raises with your feet at different angles. You can easily target the inner part of your calves by moving your toes away from each other to form a right angle (or more) with your feet. You will target the outer part of your calves if you move your toes toward each other so that you look pigeon-toed.

Step 5: Perform calf raises with the balls of your feet on a raised surface so that your heels are unsupported. This allows you to exercise your calves throughout their entire range of motion.

Abdominal exercises (see previous descriptions of these exercises)

1) *Sit ups with inflatable ball*—70 reps plus a twist. As you sit up and crunch, twist your torso to the left, then twist to the right, and lie back down. This is one rep.

2) *Leg lifts*—60 reps

3) *Bicycles*—3 sets of 25

4) *Abdominal crunch*—3 sets of 20 reps

5) *Vertical leg crunch*—3 sets of 20 reps

More Health and Fitness Resources from Harvest House Publishers

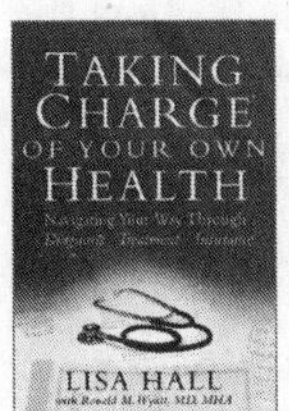

Taking Charge of Your Own Health
Navigating Your Way Through Diagnosis, Treatment, Insurance
Lisa Hall, with Ronald M. Wyatt, MD, MHA

When you face a health-care need today, you have to be prepared for less personal attention, more complications with insurance and government programs, and a *40 percent misdiagnosis rate*, according to recent national surveys.

Lisa Hall's years-long search for diagnosis has given her top-to-bottom experience with the health-care system. Aided by the expertise of internal-medicine doctor Ronald Wyatt, Lisa provides a wide variety of practical guidance on how to find the right doctor, navigate medical insurance, and avoid being a victim of hospital mistakes.

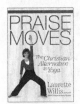

Praise Moves: The Christian Alternative to Yoga (DVD)
Laurette Willis

Would you like to increase your flexibility, improve your circulation, and enhance your level of energy? Finally there's a program that offers proven stretching and flexibility exercises without troubling Eastern influences. Now you can fill your mind with the Word of God as you practice the postures on this DVD that will promote healing, relieve stress, and enhance relaxation.

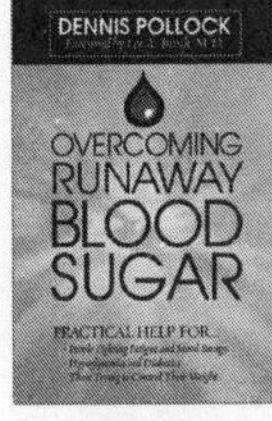

Overcoming Runaway Blood Sugar
Dennis Pollock

With this positive, can-do approach, you can gain maximum health while losing excess pounds. You'll discover why runaway blood sugar is a key factor in food cravings and weight issues, reasons and motivation to change your lifestyle, and diet and exercise that really work.

Whether you are diabetic, have a family history of diabetes, or are simply tired of being sick and tired, *Overcoming Runaway Blood Sugar* may very well change the way you view eating and exercise forever.

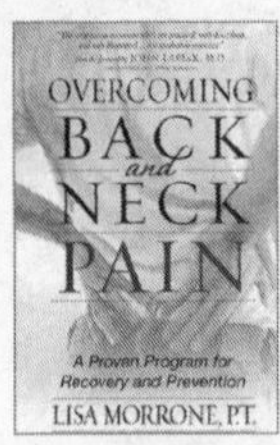

Overcoming Back and Neck Pain

A Proven Program for Recovery and Prevention

Lisa Morrone, PT

Physical therapist Lisa Morrone gives you a way to say *no* to the treadmill of prescriptions, endless treatments, and a limited lifestyle. This straightforward, clinically proven approach offers the most effective exercises, guidelines, and lifestyle adjustments for back and neck problems, showing you how to benefit from good posture and "core stability," strengthen and stretch key muscles, and recover from pain caused by compressed or degenerated discs.

With Lisa's help, you can gain freedom from pain—and *regain* your freedom to enjoy work, friends, family, and a fulfilling life.

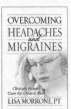

Overcoming Headaches and Migraines

Clinically Proven Cure for Chronic Pain

Lisa Morrone, PT

If you're one of the millions who experience chronic or debilitating headaches and are looking for practical help and answers, physical therapist Lisa Morrone has them. Nearly 20 years of teaching, research, and hands-on treatment have given her a thorough, broad-based perspective on head pain.

As a headache or migraine sufferer, you don't have to resign yourself to being a pill-popping victim. This comprehensive resource combines effective habits, exercises, and lifestyle adjustments to help you end head-pain disability and get back a life you can enjoy and share.